Clear & Simple Medical English in Dialogues:

Vocabulary For ESL Health Care Professionals

Jackie Bolen

www.eslspeaking.org

Table of Contents

About the Author: Jackie Bolen

I taught English in South Korea for 10 years to every level and type of student. I've taught every age from kindergarten kids to adults. I now live and teach in Vancouver, Canada.

In case you were wondering what my academic qualifications are, I hold a Master of Arts in Psychology. During my time in Korea, I completed both the Cambridge CELTA and DELTA certification programs. With the combination of almost ten years teaching ESL/EFL learners of all ages and levels, and the more formal teaching qualifications I've obtained, I have a solid foundation on which to offer advice to English learners.

Please send me an email with any questions or feedback that you might have.

YouTube: www.youtube.com/c/jackiebolen

Pinterest: www.pinterest.com/eslspeaking

ESL Speaking: www.eslspeaking.org

Email: jb.business.online@gmail.com

You might also be interested in these books (by Jackie Bolen):

- Short Stories in English for Intermediate Learners

- Master English Collocations in 15 Minutes a Day

- IELTS Academic Vocabulary Builder

Please also join my email list. You'll get helpful tips, ideas and resources for learning English, delivered straight to your inbox each week: www.eslspeaking.org/learn-english.

Introduction to Medical English Dialogues

Welcome to this book designed to help you expand your knowledge of medical English. My goal is to help you speak more fluently and understand more of what you hear.

Let's face it, English can be difficult to master, even for the best students. In this book, you'll find dialogues that are ideal for intermediate-level students.

The best way to learn new vocabulary is in context.

To get the most bang for your buck, be sure to do the following:

- Review frequently.

- Try to use some of the phrases and expressions in real life.

- Don't be nervous about making mistakes. That's how you'll get better at English!

- Consider studying with a friend so you can help each other stay motivated.

- Use a notebook and write down new words, idioms, expressions, etc. that you run across. Review frequently so that they stay fresh in your mind.

- Be sure to answer the questions at the end of each dialogue. I recommend trying to do this from memory. No peeking!

- I recommend doing one dialogue a day. This will be more beneficial than finishing the entire book in a week or two.

Good luck and I wish you well on your journey to becoming more proficient with medical English.

How are you Feeling?

A nurse and patient are discussing a few things.

Nurse: Good morning! I'll be your nurse today. How are you **feeling?**

Patient: I'm doing okay, I guess. A bit tired, but that's to be expected, right?

Nurse: Absolutely, it's completely normal to feel a bit fatigued. Can you tell me how your **pain levels** are?

Patient: It's **manageable**. The **medication** helps, but there's still some discomfort.

Nurse: We'll keep an eye on that and adjust your pain management accordingly. Have you been able to get some **rest**?

Patient: Not much, to be honest. It's hard to sleep in here with all the beeping machines and the constant activity.

Nurse: I understand. Hospital environments can be challenging for getting quality sleep. We'll see if there's anything we can do to make it more comfortable for you. How about your **appetite**? Have you been able to eat?

Patient: Not really. The food is okay, but I just don't have much of an appetite.

Nurse: It's common for appetite to decrease after a procedure. Have you been experiencing any nausea or dizziness?

Patient: No, none of that so far. Just the soreness and a bit of headache.

Nurse: That's good to hear. We'll monitor your **symptoms** closely. Now, let's talk about your mobility. Have you been able to get up and move around a bit?

Patient: I've been afraid to overdo it. The doctor did mention taking it easy for a while.

Nurse: That's understandable. We'll start with some gentle exercises to prevent stiffness and promote **circulation.** And don't hesitate to use the call button if you need anything at all. How about any **concerns** or questions you might have?

Patient: Well, I was wondering about the **recovery process**. How long do they expect me to stay in the hospital?

Nurse: It depends on how well you progress. If all goes well, maybe a few days.

Vocabulary

circulation: The movement of blood through the body, facilitated by the heart and blood vessels.

concerns: Worries or anxieties about something.

feeling: The state of one's physical or emotional condition.

pain levels: The degree or intensity of discomfort experienced by a person.

manageable: Capable of being handled, controlled, or regulated.

medication: A substance, often in the form of a drug, used to treat, cure, or relieve symptoms of a medical condition.

rest: The act of ceasing physical activity and relaxing.

appetite: The desire or willingness to eat.

symptoms: Indications or manifestations of a medical condition or disease.

recovery process: The series of steps and stages involved in returning to a normal or healthier state after an illness or medical procedure.

Vocabulary Challenge

1. After surgery, patients are advised to get plenty of _____ to aid in the healing process.

2. If you experience persistent _____ such as fatigue or dizziness, it's essential to consult with a healthcare professional.

3. Managing stress and maintaining a healthy lifestyle can positively impact _____.

4. It's crucial to communicate any _____ or issues related to your treatment plan with your healthcare provider.

5. The doctor prescribed a new _____ to help control the symptoms of the chronic condition.

6. Adequate _____ is essential for the body to repair itself and for overall well-being.

7. Patients recovering from surgery need to follow a structured _____ to ensure a smooth return to normal functioning.

8. _____ is a common concern for individuals managing chronic pain conditions.

9. Maintaining a balanced diet is crucial for overall health and can positively impact your _____.

Answers:

1. rest
2. symptoms
3. circulation
4. concerns
5. medication
6. rest
7. recovery process
8. pain levels
9. appetite

Comprehension Questions

1. How does the patient describe their overall feeling to the nurse?

2. What is the patient's response regarding their pain levels, and how does the nurse plan to address it?

3. Why has the patient found it challenging to get quality sleep in the hospital?

4. How does the nurse respond to the patient's lack of appetite, and what information does the patient provide about their eating habits?

5. Besides soreness and a headache, what other symptoms does the patient mention, and how does the nurse react?

6. Why has the patient been hesitant to get up and move around, and how does the nurse plan to address this concern?

7. What does the nurse suggest regarding mobility and preventing stiffness in the patient?

8. What aspect of the recovery process does the patient express concern about, and how does the nurse respond?

9. According to the nurse, how long might the patient expect to stay in the hospital, and what factor does it depend on?

10. How does the nurse conclude the dialogue, ensuring the patient feels supported and informed?

Answers

1. The patient describes feeling okay but a bit tired.

2. The patient states that their pain is manageable, and the nurse plans to monitor and adjust pain management accordingly.

3. The patient finds it challenging to sleep due to the beeping machines and constant activity in the hospital.

4. The nurse acknowledges the decreased appetite after a procedure and asks if the patient has experienced any nausea or dizziness.

5. The patient mentions only soreness and a bit of a headache, and the nurse reacts positively, stating they will monitor the symptoms closely.

6. The patient has been afraid to overdo it, and the nurse plans to start with gentle exercises to prevent stiffness and promote circulation.

7. The nurse suggests starting with gentle exercises to prevent stiffness and promote circulation.

8. The patient expresses concern about the recovery process and asks how long they might stay in the hospital. The nurse responds that it depends on how well they progress, maybe a few days.

9. According to the nurse, the patient might expect to stay in the hospital for a few days, depending on how well they progress.

10. The nurse concludes by reassuring the patient they will monitor closely, suggesting gentle exercises, and encouraging the use of the call button for any needs.

Discussion Questions

1. How does the nurse establish a positive and comforting atmosphere in the initial interaction with the patient?

2. In what ways can healthcare professionals effectively address and manage a patient's discomfort while ensuring their well-being?

3. Why is it important for the nurse to inquire about symptoms like nausea and dizziness, even if the patient hasn't experienced them?

4. Discuss the challenges a patient may face regarding mobility after a medical procedure. How can healthcare providers strike a balance between encouraging movement and preventing overexertion?

5. Discuss the importance of open communication between healthcare providers and patients, as demonstrated in the dialogue. How does it contribute to patient comfort and understanding?

6. Reflect on the nurse's response regarding the expected duration of the patient's stay. How might this information positively impact the patient's mindset and recovery journey?

Persistent Headaches

A patient is talking to his doctor about a problem.

Patient: Good morning, Doctor. I've been experiencing some **persistent headaches** lately, and it's starting to worry me.

Doctor: Good morning! I'm sorry to hear that. When did the headaches start, and have you noticed any specific patterns or **triggers**?

Patient: They began about two weeks ago, and it feels like they're mostly around my temples. I can't pinpoint any specific triggers, but they're becoming more frequent.

Doctor: I see. Any other symptoms like **nausea**, **dizziness**, or changes in vision?

Patient: No. It's just the headaches that bother me. I've been taking **over-the-counter** pain relievers, but they only provide temporary relief.

Doctor: Chronic headaches can be concerning. Let's talk about your medical history. Have you had any recent changes in your lifestyle, stress levels, or sleep patterns?

Patient: Well, work has been more demanding lately, and I've noticed that I'm not getting as much sleep as I used to. Stress has definitely been higher.

Doctor: Stress and **sleep deprivation** can indeed contribute to headaches. We'll address that. I recommend a thorough examination and, possibly, some **diagnostic tests**. In the meantime, let's discuss strategies to manage stress and improve your sleep.

Patient: That sounds like a good plan. I'm willing to try anything.

Doctor: Great! I'll schedule some **imaging tests** to rule out any underlying issues. Meanwhile, keep a headache diary noting when they occur, what you eat, and your activities before the headaches. It'll help us identify potential triggers.

Patient: Sure, I'll start keeping track. I appreciate your help, Doctor.

Doctor: My pleasure. We'll get to the bottom of this. If the headaches worsen or new symptoms arise, don't hesitate to contact me.

Patient: Thank you, Doctor.

Vocabulary

headaches: Pain in the head, often characterized by aching or throbbing sensations.

triggers: Factors or events that can cause or contribute to the occurrence of headaches.

persistent: Continuing for a long time or recurring frequently.

nausea: A feeling of discomfort or unease in the stomach, often leading to the urge to vomit.

dizziness: A sensation of lightheadedness or unsteadiness.

over-the-counter: Medications that can be purchased without a prescription.

chronic: Persisting for a long time or occurring frequently.

diagnostic tests: Examinations or procedures conducted to identify the cause of a medical issue.

sleep deprivation: Not getting enough sleep or experiencing a lack of quality sleep.

imaging tests: Procedures that use various technologies to create visual representations of the inside of the body.

Vocabulary Challenge

1. She has been experiencing _____for weeks, and it's affecting her daily life.
2. Identifying the _____of your headaches is essential to find effective treatment.
3. The patient reported _____stomach discomfort after taking the prescribed medication.
4. After the accident, he felt a sense of _____and had to sit down to regain his balance.
5. You can find some _____pain relievers at the pharmacy to help with the headaches.
6. _____use of certain medications can lead to adverse effects on health.
7. The doctor recommended a series of _____to understand the cause of the mysterious symptoms.
8. _____is a common side effect of irregular sleep patterns and can impact overall well-being.

9. _____such as X-rays and MRIs are valuable tools in diagnosing internal health conditions.

Answers:

1. headaches
2. triggers
3. nausea
4. dizziness
5. over-the-counter
6. chronic
7. diagnostic tests
8. sleep deprivation
9. imaging tests

Comprehension Questions

1. When did the patient's headaches start, and where does it feel like they are mostly located?

2. What specific symptoms is the doctor inquiring about besides headaches, and how does the patient respond?

3. What measures has the patient taken to alleviate the headaches, and what has been the outcome?

4. According to the doctor, what can chronic headaches potentially indicate, and what aspects of the patient's history are explored to understand the possible causes?

5. How does the patient describe recent changes in their lifestyle, and what factors related to work and sleep patterns does the patient mention?

6. In response to the patient's acknowledgment of stress and sleep deprivation, what approach does the doctor propose to address these contributing factors?

7. What is the doctor's recommendation concerning diagnostic tests, and what additional strategies are discussed to manage stress and improve sleep?

8. How does the patient express their willingness to cooperate with the suggested strategies?

9. What specific action does the doctor plan, and what information does the patient agree to keep track of in a diary?

10. How does the doctor conclude the dialogue, ensuring the patient feels supported and informed about future steps?

Answers:

1. The patient's headaches began about two weeks ago, and they feel like they're mostly around the temples.

2. The doctor inquires about symptoms like nausea, dizziness, or changes in vision. The patient responds that there are no other symptoms; it's just the headaches that bother them.

3. The patient has been taking over-the-counter pain relievers, but they only provide temporary relief.

4. Chronic headaches can be concerning, and the doctor explores recent changes in the patient's lifestyle, stress levels, and sleep patterns.

5. The patient mentions that work has been more demanding lately, and they're not getting as much sleep as they used to due to higher stress.

6. The doctor proposes a thorough examination and diagnostic tests to address the potential causes of chronic headaches.

7. The doctor recommends keeping a headache diary and discusses strategies to manage stress and improve sleep.

8. The patient expresses willingness to try anything to address the headaches.

9. The doctor plans to schedule imaging tests, and the patient agrees to keep a headache diary noting when they occur, what they eat, and their activities before the headaches.

10. The doctor concludes by assuring the patient they'll get to the bottom of the issue and encourages them to contact if headaches worsen or new symptoms arise.

Discussion Questions

1. Why is it important for the doctor to inquire about symptoms like nausea, dizziness, or changes in vision, even if the patient hasn't experienced them?

2. Discuss the limitations of relying on over-the-counter pain relievers for chronic headaches. What could be potential drawbacks or risks?

3. Explore the impact of increased work demands and reduced sleep on an individual's overall well-being. How might these factors contribute to chronic headaches?

4. Discuss the significance of keeping a headache diary. How might it help in identifying potential triggers and contributing factors?

5. Reflect on the doctor's assurance to the patient and the encouragement to contact if headaches worsen or new symptoms arise. Why is ongoing communication important in managing healthcare concerns?

Test Results

Jess and her doctor are discussing some test results.

Doctor: How are you feeling today? A bit better I hope?

Jess: Yes, definitely. I haven't felt **nauseous** since I switched the medication.

Doctor: Okay good. I have your test results here.

Jess: Is it good news or bad news?

Doctor: Well, a bit of both. You'll need **surgery** to remove the **tumour** in your leg. However, the **biopsy** showed that it's **benign**.

Jess: Benign? Isn't that bad?

Doctor: Oh no. Sorry for using **doctor jargon**. It's not **cancerous**. But we should remove it because it's getting bigger and will soon make it more difficult for you to play soccer and do other stuff like that.

Jess: Okay. That's good news then. When can I get the surgery?

Doctor: Please talk to the receptionist after our appointment. She'll give the **surgeon** a call and get you all set up. It's usually a 2-3 month wait for less urgent situations like yours.

Jess: Okay. Thank you.

Vocabulary

nauseous: Feeling sick to your stomach, like you might throw up (vomit).

surgery: A procedure on the body, usually involves cutting under the skin, or into another part of the body (the eye for example).

tumour: A mass or growth inside the body that shouldn't be there. Can be cancerous, or not.

biopsy: Removing a small sample of tissue from inside the body to do tests on (usually for cancer).

benign: Not cancerous or dangerous.

doctor jargon: Words that doctors use which patients don't understand.

cancerous: Describes something that has cancer cells.

surgeon: A person who does surgery.

Vocabulary Challenge

1. I need to book an appointment with the _____ but she's booked up for months because of Covid delays.

2. I just found out that I have a _____ in my stomach. I have to wait and see if it's cancerous, or not.

3. I'm so relieved. My doctor just let me know that my tumour is _____.

4. I have a lump on my arm. I hope it's not _____ but I'm scared to go to the doctor and find out.

5. I'm scheduled for _____ on May 29th and 7:00 in the morning. Can you take me?

6. I have to get a _____ on this tumour to find out if it's cancerous. I hope it isn't.

7. My son always gets _____ when riding in a car.

Answers:

1. surgeon

2. tumour

3. benign

4. cancerous

5. surgery

6. biopsy

7. nauseous

Comprehension Questions

1. How has Jess been feeling since she switched her medication?

2. What does the doctor reveal about Jess's test results?

3. What is the doctor's recommendation regarding the tumor in Jess's leg?

4. What does "benign" mean in the context of the biopsy results?

5. Why does the doctor suggest removing the tumor despite it being benign?

6. How does Jess react when she hears that the tumor is not cancerous?

7. What concerns does Jess express about the tumor, prompting the need for surgery?

8. What information does the doctor provide about the timeline for Jess's surgery?

9. What is Jess's response to the news about the surgery timeline?

10. Who does the doctor suggest Jess speak to regarding scheduling the surgery?

Answers:

1. Jess has been feeling better since she switched her medication.

2. The doctor reveals that Jess will need surgery to remove the benign tumor in her leg.

3. The doctor recommends removing the tumor because it's getting bigger and may affect Jess's ability to engage in physical activities.

4. In this context, "benign" means that the tumor is not cancerous.

5. The doctor suggests removing the tumor because it's growing and may impact Jess's ability to play sports like soccer.

6. Jess reacts positively when she learns that the tumor is not cancerous, saying, "Okay. That's good news then."

7. Jess expresses concerns about the tumor getting bigger and affecting her ability to play soccer and other activities.

8. The doctor mentions that it's usually a 2-3 month wait for less urgent situations like Jess's surgery.

9. Jess responds with "Okay. Thank you" when informed about the surgery timeline.

10. The doctor suggests Jess speak to the receptionist after the appointment to schedule the surgery.

Discussion Questions

1. What does the term "benign" mean in the context of the dialogue, and how does the doctor explain it to Jess?

2. How does Jess feel about the news that she needs surgery, and why is the doctor recommending the surgery?

3. What role does the receptionist play in the process, and why is it important for Jess to speak to her after the appointment?

4. How might the news of needing surgery impact Jess's daily life and activities, especially her involvement in sports like soccer?

5. What emotions and thoughts might Jess be experiencing as she processes the information about the surgery and the benign tumor?

Arthritis

A patient is talking to his doctor about joint pain.

Doctor: Good morning! I'm Dr. Thompson. How can I assist you today?

Patient: Hi, Dr. Thompson. I've been experiencing **joint pain** and **stiffness**, especially in my hands and knees. I'm wondering if it could be **arthritis.**

Doctor: I see. I'm sorry to hear about your discomfort. When did you first notice the joint pain, and have you observed any swelling or **redness**?

Patient: It started a few months ago, and yes, there's some **swelling,** particularly in my fingers. The pain is worse in the mornings.

Doctor: **Morning stiffness** is a common symptom. Have you noticed if the pain and stiffness improve as the day goes on or if they persist throughout?

Patient: It tends to get better as the day progresses, but it's still there to some extent.

Doctor: Okay. Besides your hands and knees, do you experience joint pain in any other areas? And have you noticed any limitations in your range of motion?

Patient: It's mostly my hands and knees, and yes, I've noticed a bit of difficulty moving them, especially after sitting for a while.

Doctor: I'd like to perform a physical examination and order some tests to get a clearer picture. Arthritis comes in various forms, so we want to identify the specific type. Additionally, we'll discuss your medical history to understand any **contributing factors.**

Patient: What are the treatment options for arthritis if that's indeed what I have?

Doctor: Treatment varies based on the type of arthritis. It might involve medications, physical therapy, and lifestyle modifications. We'll tailor a plan to manage your symptoms and improve your overall joint health.

Patient: I've heard about arthritis diets and supplements. Do those help?

Doctor: Dietary changes and supplements can play a role, and we can discuss those as part of a **comprehensive approach**. However, it's crucial to determine the specific type of arthritis before recommending specific interventions.

Vocabulary

joint pain: Discomfort or soreness in the areas where two or more bones meet.

stiffness: The resistance or difficulty in moving joints, often accompanied by discomfort.

arthritis: Inflammation of the joints, leading to pain, swelling, and stiffness.

swelling: Abnormal enlargement or puffiness in a body part, often due to fluid accumulation.

redness: The appearance of a reddish color, indicating increased blood flow or inflammation.

morning stiffness: A sensation of joint tightness and reduced mobility, particularly experienced in the morning.

contributing factors: Elements or conditions that have an impact on a particular situation, in this case, factors influencing joint health.

comprehensive approach: A holistic and thorough strategy that addresses various aspects of a condition or situation.

Vocabulary Challenge

1. After sitting for a while, the patient noticed _____in the joints of their hands and knees.

2. The doctor recommended a _____to manage the patient's arthritis symptoms, involving medications and lifestyle modifications.

3. _____makes it difficult for me to play sports.

4. _____is the resistance or difficulty in moving joints, which can be a common experience with arthritis.

5. _____is a sensation of joint tightness and reduced mobility, especially felt in the morning.

6. _____is the appearance of a reddish color, indicating increased blood flow or inflammation in the joints.

7. _____are elements or conditions that may influence joint health, and the doctor will consider them during the examination.

Answers:

1. swelling

2. comprehensive approach

3. joint pain/arthritis

4. stiffness

5. morning stiffness

6. redness

7. contributing factors

Comprehension Questions

1. Who is the doctor in this dialogue?

2. What symptoms does the patient describe experiencing?

3. How long has the patient been dealing with joint pain?

4. Describe the patient's experience with morning stiffness.

5. Which areas of the body does the patient mention having joint pain?

6. What does the doctor suggest to understand the specific type of arthritis?

7. How does the patient describe the progression of pain and stiffness throughout the day?

8. What is the doctor's approach to addressing the patient's symptoms?

9. What are some potential treatment options for arthritis mentioned by the doctor?

Answers:

1. The doctor's name is Dr. Thompson.

2. The patient is experiencing joint pain and stiffness.

3. The patient first noticed the joint pain a few months ago.

4. Morning stiffness is a common symptom, and the pain tends to improve as the day progresses but remains to some extent.

5. The patient experiences joint pain mostly in the hands and knees.

6. The doctor would like to perform a physical examination and order tests to identify the specific type of arthritis.

7. The pain tends to improve throughout the day but remains to some extent.

8. Treatment for arthritis varies based on the specific type and may involve medications, physical therapy, and lifestyle modifications.

9. Treatment for arthritis varies based on the specific type and may involve medications, physical therapy, and lifestyle modifications.

Discussion Questions

1. What are some common symptoms of arthritis, and how do they impact a person's daily life?

2. In what ways can morning stiffness be challenging for individuals with arthritis, and how might it influence their daily routines?

3. How does the doctor approach the diagnosis of arthritis, and why is it important to identify the specific type?

4. What are some of the treatment options mentioned by the doctor for managing arthritis, and how do they vary based on the type of arthritis?

5. How can individuals with arthritis adapt their lifestyles to improve joint health and reduce the impact of symptoms?

Some Bad News

A doctor is telling her patient that he has cancer.

Doctor: Good afternoon, Mr. Johnson. I've reviewed your test results, and I'm afraid I have some difficult news to share.

Patient: Oh, okay. What is it?

Doctor: I wish I could say it was better news, but the tests indicate that you have a form of advanced cancer. I understand this is a lot to take in . . .

Patient: **Cancer**? I... I never expected to hear something like that. What does this mean?

Doctor: I know this is overwhelming. The type of cancer you have is **aggressive**, and we'll need to discuss **treatment options**. We'll explore chemotherapy, radiation, and possibly surgery. It's important to start treatment as soon as possible.

Patient: I...I don't even know what to say. What are my chances?

Doctor: Cancer can develop for various reasons. We'll work together to understand your medical history. As for your chances, I'll be honest; the **prognosis** is not that optimistic. However, we'll focus on providing the best care possible to improve your **quality of life**.

Patient: This is a lot to process. What about my family? How do I tell them?

Doctor: It's essential to have a **support system**, and involving your family is crucial. We can arrange a meeting with them to discuss the **diagnosis**, treatment options, and what to expect moving forward. Additionally, we have counseling services available.

Patient: I never thought I'd be facing something like this. What about my job? My life?

Doctor: We'll **collaborate** with you to create a treatment plan that considers your overall **well-being**. It's common for cancer treatment to impact daily life, including work. We can discuss potential **adjustments** and accommodations.

Patient: I appreciate your honesty. What's the next step?

Doctor: In the coming days, we'll schedule further tests to gather more detailed information about the cancer. Our oncology team will then formulate a comprehensive treatment plan tailored to your specific situation.

Patient: I guess we'll take it one step at a time.

Vocabulary

prognosis: The likely course or outcome of a medical condition, especially the chance of recovery.

diagnosis: The identification of a disease or medical condition through examination and analysis of symptoms and test results.

treatment options: Different approaches or methods available for managing and addressing a medical condition, such as chemotherapy, radiation, or surgery.

cancer: A group of diseases characterized by the uncontrolled growth and spread of abnormal cells in the body.

aggressive (cancer): Refers to a type of cancer that tends to grow and spread rapidly.

support system: A network of people who provide emotional, practical, and sometimes financial assistance during challenging times.

well-being: The state of being comfortable, healthy, or happy, especially in terms of one's overall health and happiness.

adjustments: Changes or modifications made to adapt to a new situation or condition.

collaborate: To work together with others in a joint intellectual effort.

quality of life: The overall well-being and satisfaction experienced by an individual in various aspects of their life, including health, happiness, and fulfillment.

Vocabulary Challenge

1. The _____ is the likely course or outcome of a medical condition, especially the chance of recovery.

2. The process of the _____ involves the identification of a disease or medical condition through examination and analysis of symptoms and test results.

3. There are various _____ available for managing and addressing a medical condition, including chemotherapy, radiation, or surgery.

4. _____ is a group of diseases characterized by the uncontrolled growth and spread of abnormal cells in the body.

5. An _____ type of cancer refers to a cancer that tends to grow and spread rapidly.

6. A _____ is a network of people who provide emotional, practical, and sometimes financial assistance during challenging times.

7. _____ is the state of being comfortable, healthy, or happy, especially in terms of one's overall health and happiness.

8. _____ are changes or modifications made to adapt to a new situation or condition.

9. To _____ is to work together with others in a joint intellectual effort.

10. _____ encompasses the overall well-being and satisfaction experienced by an individual in various aspects of their life, including health, happiness, and fulfillment.

Answers:

1. prognosis

2. diagnosis

3. treatment options

4. cancer

5. aggressive

6. support system

7. well-being

8. adjustments

9. collaborate

10. quality of life

Comprehension Questions

1. What did the doctor find during the test results review?

2. What is the difficult news the doctor shared with the patient?

3. How does the doctor describe the type of cancer the patient has?

4. What treatment options does the doctor mention for the aggressive cancer?

5. What is the patient's initial response upon learning about the cancer diagnosis?

6. Why does the doctor mention that cancer can develop for various reasons?

7. How does the doctor suggest involving the patient's family in the situation?

8. What aspect of the patient's life does the doctor acknowledge may be impacted by cancer treatment?

Answers

1. The doctor found that the patient has a form of advanced cancer.

2. The difficult news is that the patient has a form of advanced cancer.

3. The doctor describes the type of cancer as aggressive.

4. The doctor mentions exploring chemotherapy, radiation, and possibly surgery as treatment options.

5. The patient expresses surprise, saying, "Cancer? I... I never expected to hear something like that. What does this mean?"

6. The doctor mentions that cancer can develop for various reasons, and sometimes it's difficult to pinpoint an exact cause.

7. The doctor suggests arranging a meeting with the patient's family to discuss the diagnosis, treatment options, and what to expect moving forward.

8. The doctor acknowledges that cancer treatment may impact daily life, including work, and mentions discussing potential adjustments and accommodations.

Discussion Questions

1. What emotions do you think the patient might be experiencing upon learning about the cancer diagnosis?

2. In what ways does the doctor convey empathy and support to the patient during the conversation?

3. What challenges do you think the patient might face in processing the information about the cancer diagnosis?

4. Why is it important for the doctor to emphasize collaboration with the patient in creating a treatment plan?

5. In your opinion, what role does open and honest communication play in the doctor-patient relationship during such difficult conversations?

My Prescription

A patient is picking up her prescription from a pharmacist.

Patient: Good afternoon. I'm here to pick up my **prescription**.

Pharmacist: Good afternoon! Sure, could you tell me your name and date of birth?

Patient: It's Sarah Thompson, born on July 15, 1985.

Pharmacist: Let me pull up your prescription. Ah, yes, I see it here. You have a **medication** for managing your blood pressure. How has it been working for you?

Patient: I've noticed some **side effects**, like dizziness. Is that normal?

Pharmacist: It's not uncommon to experience side effects with certain medications. Dizziness can be one of them. Have you been taking the medication with food?

Patient: Yes, I take it with my breakfast every day.

Pharmacist: That's good. Taking it with food can help minimize some side effects. However, if the dizziness persists or becomes severe, I recommend speaking with your doctor. They might adjust the **dosage** or consider an alternative medication.

Patient: Alright, I'll keep an eye on it. Also, I've been having trouble remembering to take it at the same time every day. Is that a problem?

Pharmacist: **Consistency** is essential for medications like this one to be most effective. If you find it challenging to remember, consider setting an alarm on your phone or associating it with another daily routine, like brushing your teeth.

Patient: I'll give it a try. Is there anything else I should know about this medication?

Pharmacist: It's essential to avoid any **interactions** with certain foods or other medications. I'll provide you with an information **leaflet** that outlines potential interactions and things to watch out for. If you have any questions, don't hesitate to ask.

Patient: One more thing – is there a **generic** version of this medication available?

Pharmacist: Yes, there is a generic alternative. It might be a more **cost-effective** option for you. I can discuss this with your doctor and make the switch if you're interested.

Patient: That sounds great. Thank you for your assistance.

Pharmacist: If you have any more questions or concerns, feel free to reach out.

Vocabulary

prescription: A written order from a doctor for a specific medication.

medication: A substance used to treat, cure, or prevent a disease or medical condition.

side effects: Unintended and often undesirable effects of a medication.

dosage: The prescribed amount of a medication to be taken.

consistency: The quality of being consistent, regular, or unchanging; in the context of medication, taking it at the same time every day.

interactions: The effects that occur when the action of one substance is affected by the presence of another substance, such as interactions between medications and foods.

generic: A term used to describe a non-brand-name version of a drug, usually less expensive than the brand-name version but with the same active ingredients.

cost-effective: Providing good value for the amount of money spent; economical.

leaflet: A small printed sheet of paper containing information or instructions.

Vocabulary Challenge

1. The doctor provided me with a _____ for antibiotics to treat my infection.
2. This _____ is recommended to alleviate the symptoms of allergies.
3. Some medications may cause _____, such as drowsiness or nausea.
4. The _____ for this painkiller is one tablet every four hours.
5. _____ is crucial when taking daily medication to ensure its effectiveness.
6. Be aware of potential drug _____ when combining different medications.
7. The _____ version of the drug is more affordable, but it works just as effectively.
8. Choosing a _____ treatment option can help manage healthcare costs.
9. The pharmacist included a helpful _____ with details about the medication's use and possible side effects.
10. To maintain _____ in your treatment, take the medication at the same time every day.

Answers

1. prescription
2. medication
3. side effects
4. dosage
5. consistency
6. interactions
7. generic
8. cost-effective
9. leaflet
10. consistency

Comprehension Questions

1. What is the patient's name and date of birth?
2. What medication is the patient picking up, and for what purpose?
3. What side effect has the patient noticed from taking the medication?
4. How does the pharmacist suggest minimizing side effects related to dizziness?
5. What recommendation does the pharmacist give if the dizziness persists or becomes severe?
6. How does the pharmacist advise the patient to maintain consistency in taking the medication?
7. Why does the pharmacist emphasize consistency in medication intake?
8. What alternative methods does the pharmacist suggest for the patient to remember to take the medication at the same time every day?
9. What does the pharmacist mention about potential interactions related to the medication?
10. What information does the pharmacist offer to provide the patient regarding potential interactions and other important details?

Answers

1. The patient's name is Sarah Thompson, and her date of birth is July 15, 1985.

2. The patient is picking up medication for managing blood pressure.

3. The patient has noticed dizziness as a side effect of the medication.

4. The pharmacist suggests minimizing side effects by taking the medication with food.

5. If the dizziness persists or becomes severe, the pharmacist recommends the patient speak with their doctor for potential dosage adjustment or consider an alternative medication.

6. To maintain consistency in taking the medication, the pharmacist advises the patient to set an alarm on their phone or associate it with another daily routine.

7. Emphasizing consistency is crucial for medications like this one to be most effective.

8. The pharmacist suggests alternative methods for the patient to remember to take the medication at the same time every day, such as setting an alarm on the phone or associating it with another daily routine, like brushing teeth.

9. It's essential to avoid interactions with certain foods or other medications.

10. The pharmacist offers to provide the patient with an information leaflet containing details about potential interactions and other important information.

Discussion Questions

1. In what ways might experiencing side effects impact a patient's adherence?

2. What are some practical strategies you use or can suggest to enhance consistency in taking medication regularly?

3. How important is it for healthcare professionals to consider the potential economic impact of medications when discussing treatment options with patients?

4. Discuss the role of education in managing potential side effects and maintaining medication consistency.

5. How might a patient's lifestyle and daily routines influence their ability to take medication consistently?

Trouble Breathing

A patient is talking to his doctor about a breathing issue.

Patient: Good morning, Dr. Johnson. I've been experiencing **difficulty breathing** lately, especially during physical activities. I'm concerned it might be **asthma.**

Doctor: I'm sorry to hear you're experiencing this. Let's discuss your symptoms. When did you first notice the breathing difficulties, and are there specific triggers or patterns?

Patient: It started a few weeks ago, and I've noticed it more when I exercise or when I'm exposed to certain allergens like dust and pollen.

Doctor: I see. Have you had any previous **respiratory issues,** or is this the first time you're experiencing such symptoms?

Patient: I've never had respiratory problems before.

Doctor: Asthma could be a possibility, but we'll need to conduct some tests to confirm. Have you noticed any coughing, **wheezing**, or chest **tightness**?

Patient: Yes, I've had occasional **coughing** and a feeling of tightness in my chest, especially after physical activities.

Doctor: Okay. I'll recommend some **pulmonary function tests** to assess your lung function. This will help us understand if asthma is indeed the cause. In the meantime, it's important to avoid triggers and monitor your symptoms.

Patient: If it is asthma, what are the treatment options? Can it be managed effectively?

Doctor: Asthma can be well-managed with the right treatment plan. Depending on the severity, we might prescribe **inhalers**, which can help open up your airways.

Patient: Are there any **long-term effects** of asthma, and will I be able to lead a normal life?

Doctor: With proper management, most people with asthma lead normal, active lives. It's important to follow your treatment plan and attend regular check-ups. We'll work together to understand your condition better and find the most effective ways to manage it. If you have any questions or concerns, don't hesitate to reach out.

Vocabulary

difficulty breathing: A sensation of discomfort or struggle when trying to take in air.

asthma: A chronic respiratory condition characterized by difficulty breathing, coughing, and chest tightness, often triggered by specific factors.

respiratory issues: Problems related to the breathing system, including conditions that affect the lungs and airways.

pulmonary function tests: Medical examinations that measure how well the lungs take in and release air, providing insights into respiratory function.

coughing: The act of expelling air from the lungs with a sudden, sharp sound.

wheezing: A high-pitched whistling sound produced during breathing.

chest tightness: A sensation of pressure or discomfort in the chest.

inhalers: Devices that deliver medication in the form of a mist or spray directly into the lungs, commonly used to relieve asthma symptoms.

long-term effects: The lasting consequences of a condition over an extended period.

Vocabulary Challenge

1. The patient reported experiencing _____ during physical activities.
2. The doctor discussed the possibility of _____ as the cause of the patient's symptoms.
3. The patient mentioned having no prior _____ before this episode.
4. The doctor recommended _____ to assess lung function.
5. The patient complained of persistent _____ after exposure to allergens.
6. The doctor asked if the patient had experienced any _____, such as a whistling sound during breathing.
7. The patient described a feeling of _____ in the chest, especially after exercise.
8. The doctor suggested using _____ as part of the treatment plan.
9. The patient inquired about the potential _____ of asthma on daily life.

Answers:

1. difficulty breathing
2. asthma
3. respiratory issues
4. pulmonary function tests
5. coughing
6. wheezing
7. chest tightness
8. inhalers
9. long-term effects

Comprehension Questions

1. Who is the patient talking to in this dialogue?
2. What is the patient's main concern about their health?
3. When did the patient first notice difficulty breathing?
4. In what situations does the patient experience more difficulty breathing?
5. Has the patient experienced any respiratory issues before?
6. What symptoms does the patient describe, besides difficulty breathing?
7. What tests does the doctor recommend to assess the patient's lung function?
8. How does the doctor suggest managing asthma if confirmed?
9. Are there any long-term effects mentioned for asthma?
10. What advice does the doctor give regarding monitoring symptoms and seeking help?

Answers:

1. The patient is talking to Dr. Johnson.
2. The patient is concerned about difficulty breathing, especially during physical activities.
3. The patient first noticed difficulty breathing a few weeks ago.
4. The patient experiences more difficulty breathing when exercising or when exposed to allergens like dust and pollen.
5. The patient has never had respiratory issues before.
6. Besides difficulty breathing, the patient experiences occasional coughing and a feeling of chest tightness.
7. The doctor recommends pulmonary function tests to assess the patient's lung function.
8. The doctor suggests managing asthma with inhalers, depending on the severity.
9. Long-term effects of asthma are not explicitly mentioned in the dialogue.
10. The doctor advises the patient to avoid triggers and monitor symptoms.

Discussion Questions

1. In what situations does the patient experience more difficulty breathing, and how might these triggers be managed or avoided?
2. Do you think the patient's lack of previous respiratory issues affects the doctor's approach to diagnosis and treatment?
3. How important is open communication between the patient and the doctor in understanding and managing respiratory issues like asthma?
4. Discuss the role of lifestyle modifications and avoiding triggers in the management of asthma, as mentioned by the doctor.
5. How might the doctor and patient work together to create an effective treatment plan for managing asthma in the long term?

A Torn ACL

A doctor is talking to a patient about his knee injury.

Doctor: Good morning, Mr. Davis. How can I help you today?

Patient: Hi, Doctor. I've been having some serious pain and **instability** in my knee lately.

Doctor: Let's take a look. Can you describe how the **injury** occurred?

Patient: Well, I was playing basketball, and I went to make a sudden turn. I heard a pop in my knee, and since then, it's been really painful.

Doctor: I'm sorry to hear that. Based on your **symptoms,** it's possible that you may have torn your ACL (**anterior cruciate ligament**).

Patient: Torn ACL? What does that mean, and how serious is it?

Doctor: The anterior cruciate ligament is a crucial ligament in your knee that helps stabilize it. A tear can lead to pain, swelling, and a feeling of instability. The **severity** varies, but a torn ACL often requires **medical attention** and sometimes **surgery.**

Patient: Surgery? That sounds serious. What are my options?

Doctor: I'll start with an examination and some imaging tests to confirm the **diagnosis.** Depending on the severity, I may recommend physical therapy to strengthen the surrounding muscles or, surgical intervention to repair the torn ligament.

Patient: How long does the **recovery** process usually take?

Doctor: Recovery time varies, but it can take several weeks to several months, depending on the extent of the injury and the chosen treatment. Physical therapy is crucial.

Patient: This is a lot to take in. How will this affect my daily life and activities?

Doctor: A torn ACL can **impact** your daily activities, especially those involving the knee. We'll work together to create a personalized treatment plan that considers your lifestyle and helps you get back to your regular activities as soon as possible.

Patient: Thank you, Doctor. What's the next step?

Doctor: I'll order some imaging tests to get a clear picture of the extent of the injury. Once we have the results, we can discuss the best course of action for your situation. Here's a **leaflet** with some more information about knee injuries.

Vocabulary

instability: Lack of stability or a feeling of unsteadiness in a particular area.

injury: Harm or damage to the body, in this context, referring to damage to the knee.

Anterior Cruciate Ligament (ACL): A crucial ligament in the knee that helps stabilize it.

symptoms: Observable signs or indications of a medical condition.

diagnosis: Determination of the nature and cause of a medical condition through examination and testing.

severity: The extent or seriousness of an injury or condition.

medical attention: Professional care or treatment provided by a healthcare provider.

surgery: Medical procedure involving operative intervention to treat a condition.

recovery: The process of returning to a normal state of health after illness or injury.

impact: The effect or influence of a torn ACL on the patient's daily activities and lifestyle.

leaflet: In this case, a small book with information about an injury.

Vocabulary Challenge

1. After the car accident, Sarah experienced _____ in her neck and back.
2. The athlete underwent _____ to repair the torn ligament in his knee.
3. The nurse carefully monitored the patient's vital signs to assess the _____ of his condition.
4. The doctor recommended immediate _____ for the patient's severe allergic reaction.
5. The x-ray revealed a fractured bone, confirming the _____ of the injury.
6. The pharmacist provided a detailed _____ outlining the medication's side effects and usage instructions.
7. I tore my _____ and needed surgery when I was 30.
8. _____ from knee surgery takes at least six months.

Answers:

1. instability
2. surgery
3. severity
4. medical attention
5. diagnosis
6. leaflet
7. ACL
8. recovery

Comprehension Questions

1. What symptoms does the patient describe to the doctor?
2. How did the patient's knee injury occur, according to his explanation?
3. What is the doctor's initial suspicion regarding the patient's knee condition?
4. How does the doctor explain the role of the anterior cruciate ligament (ACL) in the knee?
5. Why does the doctor mention the possibility of surgery, and how does the patient react to this suggestion?
6. What are the potential options the doctor discusses for treating a torn ACL?
7. According to the doctor, what factors influence the recovery time for a torn ACL?
8. How does the doctor reassure the patient about the impact of the injury on his daily life and activities?
9. What does the doctor suggest as the next step in diagnosing and addressing the knee injury?
10. How does the doctor emphasize a personalized approach in creating a treatment plan for the patient?

Answers

1. The patient describes serious pain and instability in the knee.

2. The patient's knee injury occurred while playing basketball, making a sudden turn, and hearing a pop in the knee.

3. The doctor suspects that the patient may have torn his ACL (anterior cruciate ligament).

4. The doctor explains that the ACL is a crucial ligament in the knee that helps stabilize it, and a tear can lead to pain, swelling, and instability.

5. The doctor mentions the possibility of surgery because a torn ACL often requires medical attention, and the patient reacts by expressing concern about the seriousness of surgery.

6. The potential options discussed for treating a torn ACL include an examination, imaging tests, physical therapy, and, in severe cases, surgical intervention.

7. The recovery time for a torn ACL varies, depending on the extent of the injury and the chosen treatment.

8. The doctor reassures the patient by stating they will work together to create a personalized treatment plan that considers his lifestyle and helps him get back to regular activities.

9. The next step is for the doctor to order imaging tests to get a clear picture of the extent of the knee injury.

10. The doctor emphasizes a personalized approach by mentioning they will discuss the best course of action based on the imaging results and create a treatment plan tailored to the patient's situation.

Discussion Questions

1. How does the doctor's approach in asking about the symptoms contribute to effective communication with the patient?

2. How does the doctor balance conveying the seriousness of the injury while maintaining a supportive tone?

3. Explore the patient's reaction to the possibility of surgery. How might a doctor address a patient's concerns and fears regarding surgical intervention?

4. Discuss the importance of a personalized treatment plan. How can tailoring the plan to the patient's lifestyle contribute to a more successful recovery?

5. Explore the emotional and psychological impact of a torn ACL on the patient's daily life and activities. How might healthcare providers support patients in coping with these challenges?

6. Consider the role of diagnostic imaging in the patient's treatment journey. How can clear imaging results influence the doctor's decision-making and the subsequent treatment plan?

Surgical Pre-Screening

A nurse is conducting a surgical pre-screening with a patient.

Nurse: Hi. I'll be conducting your surgical **pre-screening**. How are you feeling?

Patient: Hi Sarah, I'm a bit nervous but overall okay.

Nurse: Completely understandable. We're here to make sure everything goes smoothly. Have there been any changes in your medical history since your last visit?

Patient: No. I've been taking my medications as prescribed.

Nurse: Now, let's discuss any allergies you may have. Have you experienced any new allergies or **adverse reactions** to medications since we last spoke?

Patient: No **allergies** or reactions. Same as before.

Nurse: Perfect. Now, let's focus on your current medications. Can you confirm the names and **dosages** of the medications you're currently taking?

Patient: I'm taking 10mg of ABC for blood pressure, and 20mg of XYZ for cholesterol.

Nurse: Have you had any recent surgeries or procedures, even minor ones?

Patient: No surgeries, just the **routine checkups** with my primary care doctor.

Nurse: Good to know. Moving on to your **lifestyle habits,** have there been any changes in your diet, exercise routine, or smoking/alcohol habits?

Patient: I've been trying to eat healthier and walk more, but no significant changes. I don't smoke, and I only have an occasional glass of wine.

Nurse: That's great to hear that you're making **positive lifestyle choices**. Do you have any questions or concerns about the surgery?

Patient: Well, I'm a bit worried about the **anesthesia** and how I'll feel afterward.

Nurse: Anesthesia is administered by trained professionals, and they will monitor you closely. You may experience some **grogginess** or drowsiness afterward.

Patient: That makes me feel a bit better. Thanks for explaining.

Nurse: We'll provide you with **pre-op instructions**, including fasting guidelines and any specific preparations. Follow those closely, and if you have any questions later on, don't hesitate to reach out to us. We're here to support you every step of the way.

Vocabulary

pre-screening: The process of evaluating a person's health or condition before a medical procedure to ensure their suitability for the procedure.

adverse reactions: Unwanted or harmful responses that a person may experience in relation to medications or treatments.

dosages: The specific amounts of medication prescribed.

allergies: An abnormal response of the immune system to a substance that is usually harmless, resulting in symptoms ranging from mild discomfort to severe reactions.

routine checkups: Regular medical examinations or appointments with healthcare professionals to monitor general health and detect potential issues early.

lifestyle habits: Personal behaviors and choices, such as diet and exercise.

anesthesia: A medical state induced to make a patient unconscious.

grogginess: A state of drowsiness or confusion.

positive lifestyle choices: Adopting habits and behaviors that contribute to overall well-being and health.

pre-op instructions: Guidelines provided before a surgical procedure, detailing necessary preparations, including fasting and specific actions to take.

Vocabulary Challenge

1. _____ involves assessing a person's health before a medical procedure to ensure they are suitable for it.

2. _____ are unwanted or harmful responses that may occur in relation to medications.

3. Please confirm the names and _____ of the medications you are currently taking.

4. _____ is an abnormal response of the immune system to a usually harmless substance, resulting in various symptoms.

5. It's essential to attend regular _____ with healthcare professionals to monitor your general health.

6. Your _____, such as diet and exercise, play a significant role in your overall well-

being.

7. _____ is induced during surgical procedures to make a patient unconscious or insensible to pain.

8. After the surgery, you may experience some _____ or confusion due to the anesthesia.

9. Making _____ like a healthy diet and regular exercise contributes to your overall well-being.

10. Before the surgery, you'll receive _____ providing instructions on necessary preparations, including fasting.

Answers:

1. pre-screening
2. adverse reactions
3. dosages
4. allergies
5. routine checkups
6. lifestyle habits
7. anesthesia
8. grogginess
9. positive lifestyle choices
10. pre-op instructions

Comprehension Questions

1. Who will be conducting the surgical pre-screening?

2. How does the patient feel about the upcoming pre-screening?

3. Why does the nurse find the patient's nervousness understandable?

4. What has the patient's medical history been like since the last visit?

5. How has the patient been managing their medications?

6. Can the patient confirm the names and dosages of their current medications?

7. Have there been any recent surgeries or procedures for the patient?

8. What routine medical checkups has the patient had?

9. What positive changes has the patient made in their lifestyle habits?

10. What concern does the patient express about the upcoming surgery?

Answers

1. A nurse will be conducting the surgical pre-screening.

2. The patient feels a bit nervous but overall okay about the upcoming pre-screening.

3. The nurse finds the patient's nervousness understandable in the context of the surgical pre-screening.

4. There haven't been any changes in the patient's medical history since the last visit.

5. The patient has been taking their medications as prescribed.

6. Yes, the patient is taking 10mg of ABC for blood pressure and 20mg of XYZ for cholesterol.

7. No, there haven't been any recent surgeries or procedures, only routine checkups with the primary care doctor.

8. The patient has had routine checkups with their primary care doctor.

9. The patient has been trying to eat healthier, walk more, and has made no significant changes to smoking or alcohol habits.

10. The patient is worried about the anesthesia and how they'll feel afterward.

Discussion Questions

1. In what ways does the patient demonstrate effective communication about their medical history and current medications?

2. What role does the nurse play in addressing the patient's concerns and ensuring they feel comfortable throughout the pre-screening process?

3. How does the dialogue emphasize the importance of lifestyle habits in relation to overall well-being and surgery preparation?

4. In what ways does the nurse encourage the patient to actively participate in their healthcare decisions and preparations for surgery?

5. What pre-op instructions and guidelines mentioned by the nurse are crucial for the patient to follow, and why?

6. Reflect on the overall patient experience during the pre-screening. What elements contribute to a positive and supportive healthcare interaction in this scenario?

Chest Pain

A patient is talking to the doctor about chest pain.

Doctor: Good afternoon. I'm Dr. Williams. Can you tell me how you're feeling right now?

Patient: I've been experiencing **intense chest pain** and **difficulty breathing.** It started last night, and it just got worse.

Doctor: I'm sorry to hear that. We'll do our best to figure out what's going on. Can you describe the nature of the chest pain? Is it constant, or does it come and go?

Patient: It's pretty **constant,** like a heavy pressure on my chest. I also feel this sharp pain when I take deep breaths.

Doctor: Given the severity of your symptoms, we need to run some tests to understand what might be causing this. We'll start with an electrocardiogram (**ECG**) to check your heart's electrical activity. We'll also do some **blood tests** and a **chest X-ray**.

Patient: I'm really scared, Dr. Williams. Could this be a heart attack?

Doctor: I understand your concerns. Chest pain can have various causes, including heart-related issues. That's why we need to investigate further. We'll do our best to get a clear picture of what's happening. In the meantime, we're going to provide you with **medication** to help **alleviate** the pain and improve your breathing.

Patient: Okay, thank you. What if it is a **heart attack**?

Doctor: If the tests indicate a heart attack, we'll take immediate steps to manage it. Our priority is your well-being. We have a dedicated team here to provide the necessary care. It's crucial that we identify the problem accurately, and I assure you we'll keep you informed every step of the way.

Patient: I appreciate your honesty, Dr. Williams. I just want to know what's happening and get the right treatment.

Vocabulary

intense: To a large degree.

chest pain: Discomfort or pain felt in the chest area.

difficulty breathing: Trouble taking in air or feeling short of breath.

constant: Continuous, without significant variation.

electrocardiogram (ECG): A test that records the electrical activity of the heart.

blood tests: Medical examinations that analyze a sample of blood to provide information about a person's health.

chest X-ray: A test that uses X-rays to visualize the structures within the chest.

medication: A substance used to treat, cure, or relieve symptoms of a medical condition.

heart attack: A sudden and sometimes fatal occurrence of coronary thrombosis, typically resulting in chest pain and other symptoms.

alleviate: To make a symptom or condition less severe or more bearable.

Vocabulary Challenge

1. After experiencing _____, the patient described it as a heavy pressure on their chest that was continuous and unchanging.

2. To understand the _____ of the symptoms, the doctor decided to run an electrocardiogram to monitor the heart's electrical activity.

3. _____ were recommended to gather more information about the patient's health.

4. The doctor explained that medication would be provided to _____ the pain and improve the patient's breathing.

5. I have _____ when my asthma flares up.

6. A _____ is a medical imaging test that uses X-rays to visualize structures within the chest, providing additional insights into the patient's condition.

7. The patient appreciated the doctor's honesty and expressed a desire to know what's happening and receive the right _____.

8. I'm worried that my dad will have a _____, with all the meat that he eats.

Answers:

1. chest pain

2. intensity

3. blood tests

4. alleviate

5. difficulty breathing

6. chest X-ray

7. treatment

8. heart attack

Comprehension Questions

1. Who is the doctor in the dialogue?

2. What symptoms does the patient describe experiencing?

3. How does the patient describe the nature of their chest pain?

4. What tests does the doctor suggest to understand the severity of the symptoms?

5. How does the doctor respond to the patient's concerns about a heart attack?

6. What medical examinations are recommended to gather more information about the patient's health?

7. How does the doctor plan to manage the patient's pain and breathing difficulties in the meantime?

8. What imaging test is mentioned that uses X-rays to visualize structures within the chest?

9. What is the patient's main concern if the tests indicate a heart attack?

10. How does the doctor assure the patient about the healthcare team's approach to managing the situation?

Answers

1. The doctor in the dialogue is Dr. Williams.
2. The patient describes experiencing intense chest pain and difficulty breathing.
3. The patient describes the nature of their chest pain as constant, like a heavy pressure on their chest, with sharp pain when taking deep breaths.
4. The doctor suggests an electrocardiogram (ECG) to check the heart's electrical activity, blood tests, and a chest X-ray.
5. The doctor responds by acknowledging the patient's concerns and expressing the need for further investigation to understand the symptoms better.
6. Blood tests and a chest X-ray are recommended to gather more information about the patient's health.
7. The doctor plans to provide medication to alleviate the pain and improve the patient's breathing.
8. The imaging test mentioned is a chest X-ray.
9. The patient's main concern if the tests indicate a heart attack is addressed by the doctor, emphasizing immediate steps for management and the dedicated healthcare team.
10. The doctor assures the patient about the healthcare team's commitment to the patient's well-being and keeping them informed every step of the way.

Discussion Questions

1. How does Dr. Williams establish a supportive and informative tone during the conversation with the patient?
2. What role do various medical tests, such as an electrocardiogram and blood tests, play in understanding the patient's condition?
3. Explore the emotional aspect of the dialogue. How does the doctor balance empathy and professionalism when addressing the patient's concerns?
4. Reflect on the doctor's decision to provide medication. How does this contribute to the overall care and well-being of the patient?

At the Dentist

A dentist is talking with a patient.

Dentist: Good morning! I'm Dr. Smith. How are you today?

Patient: Hello, Dr. Smith. I'm doing okay, but I've been having this **persistent toothache** lately, and I thought it would be best to get it checked.

Dentist: I'm sorry to hear that you're experiencing **discomfort**. Let's take a look. When did the toothache start, and have you noticed anything specific **triggering** it?

Patient: It started about a week ago, and it seems to get worse when I eat or drink something cold. It's on the right side, towards the back.

Dentist: Thank you for sharing that information. I'll perform a **thorough** examination to identify the cause. While I'm checking, have you had any recent changes in your **oral hygiene** routine or dietary habits?

Patient: Not really, I've been brushing and flossing regularly.

Dentist: Okay, noted. I'll keep that in mind. Now, let's have a look. It appears there's some sensitivity, and I see a small **cavity**. Does the pain linger after you've finished eating?

Patient: Yes, it does. What do we need to do about it?

Dentist: I recommend filling the cavity to prevent further decay and alleviate the pain. It's a straightforward **procedure**, and we can schedule it for you. Additionally, I'll provide some recommendations for tooth sensitivity.

Patient: Sounds good, Dr. Smith. When can we schedule the procedure?

Dentist: How about next Tuesday at 2 PM? Does that work for you?

Patient: Tuesday works for me.

Dentist: You're welcome! Before you go, I'll provide a prescription for a toothpaste that might help with sensitivity.

Vocabulary

toothache: A pain or discomfort in or around a tooth.

persistent: Continuing or enduring for an extended period.

discomfort: A state of feeling uneasy or uneasy.

triggering: Causing or initiating a particular reaction or response.

thorough: Complete and detailed, leaving no part unnoticed.

oral hygiene: Care and maintenance of the mouth, teeth, and gums.

cavity: A hole or hollow space, in this context, referring to tooth decay.

procedure: A series of actions or steps taken to achieve a particular end, in this case, a dental treatment.

Vocabulary Challenge

1. The patient visited the dentist due to a _____ that had been bothering them for the past week.

2. Despite the _____ toothache, the patient continued with their daily activities.

3. The dentist performed a _____ examination to identify the cause of the discomfort.

4. The patient mentioned that the toothache seemed to get worse when they consumed something cold, _____ the pain.

5. The dentist asked about any recent changes in the patient's _____ routine or dietary habits.

6. The dentist discovered a small _____ during the examination, indicating tooth decay.

7. The patient agreed to the recommended _____ and asked when they could schedule it.

Answers

1. toothache

2. persistent

3. thorough

4. triggering

5. oral hygiene

6. cavity

7. procedure

Comprehension Questions

1. Who is the dentist in the dialogue, and how does he greet the patient?

2. What symptoms does the patient describe to Dr. Smith?

3. When did the patient's toothache start, and what seems to worsen it?

4. What specific questions does Dr. Smith ask about the patient's oral hygiene and dietary habits?

5. What does Dr. Smith discover during the examination, and what recommendation does he make to the patient?

6. How does the patient respond to Dr. Smith's recommendation, and when do they schedule the procedure?

7. What additional step does Dr. Smith take to address the patient's tooth sensitivity?

8. How does the patient express their agreement with the proposed procedure and the scheduled appointment?

9. What day and time does Dr. Smith suggest for the procedure, and how does the patient respond?

10. What does Dr. Smith offer to the patient before they leave the dental office?

Answers

1. The dentist in the dialogue is Dr. Smith, and he greets the patient by saying, "Good morning!"

2. The patient describes a persistent toothache to Dr. Smith.

3. The patient's toothache started about a week ago and worsens when eating or drinking something cold.

4. Dr. Smith asks if there have been any recent changes in the patient's oral hygiene routine or dietary habits.

5. During the examination, Dr. Smith discovers sensitivity and a small cavity. He recommends filling the cavity to prevent further decay and alleviate the pain.

6. The patient agrees to Dr. Smith's recommendation, and they schedule the procedure for next Tuesday at 2 PM.

7. Dr. Smith offers a prescription for a toothpaste to address tooth sensitivity.

8. The patient expresses agreement with the proposed procedure and the scheduled appointment by saying, "Tuesday works for me."

9. Dr. Smith suggests next Tuesday at 2 PM for the procedure, and the patient responds positively.

10. Dr. Smith offers a prescription for a toothpaste that might help with sensitivity before the patient leaves the dental office.

Discussion Questions

1. How do you typically feel about going to the dentist? Are you more anxious or comfortable, and why?

2. What factors contribute to people avoiding or delaying dental check-ups, and how can these concerns be addressed?

3. Discuss the role of preventive dental care, such as regular check-ups and cleanings, in maintaining oral health.

4. Share any positive or negative experiences you've had with dental procedures. How did the dentist contribute to your overall experience?

5. Explore the impact of dental health on overall well-being. How can maintaining good oral health contribute to a person's overall health?

A Sinus Infection

A doctor is talking to a patient who may have a sinus infection.

Doctor: Good morning! How can I help you today?

Patient: Hi, Doctor. I've been feeling really **congested** lately, and I have this constant **pressure** in my face. I'm also dealing with a lot of **nasal discharge**.

Doctor: How long have you been experiencing these issues?

Patient: It's been about a week now. At first, I thought it might be a cold, but it hasn't improved, and the pressure in my face is getting more uncomfortable.

Doctor: I see. Have you noticed any other **symptoms**, such as facial pain or headaches?

Patient: Yeah, I've had some headaches, especially around my forehead and eyes. My sense of smell is not what it used to be either.

Doctor: Those are common symptoms of a **sinus infection.** Have you had a fever or any dental pain?

Patient: No fever, but I have had a bit of **dental discomfort**, especially in my upper teeth.

Doctor: I'll proceed with a **physical examination** to check for signs of a sinus infection. I'll also recommend a **nasal endoscopy** to get a closer look inside your nasal passages.

Patient: Sure, that sounds good. What can we do to treat this if it is a sinus infection?

Doctor: If it is indeed a sinus infection, I may prescribe a course of antibiotics to target the underlying bacterial infection. Additionally, I'll recommend **decongestants** and saline nasal irrigation to help alleviate your symptoms. Stay hydrated and get lots of rest as well.

Patient: Got it. Are there any home remedies I can try in the meantime?

Doctor: Warm compresses on your face can help relieve the pressure, and over-the-counter pain relievers can ease any discomfort. Using a **humidifier** may also help.

Vocabulary

congested: Blocked or obstructed, especially in the case of nasal passages being filled with excess mucus.

pressure: The force or weight exerted on a surface.

nasal discharge: The flow of mucus from the nose, commonly known as a runny nose.

symptoms: Indications or signs of a medical condition, such as pain or headaches.

sinus infection: Inflammation or infection of the sinuses, typically caused by bacteria, viruses, or allergies.

dental discomfort: Pain or unease related to the teeth or gums.

physical examination: A thorough inspection of the body by a healthcare professional to assess signs and symptoms.

nasal endoscopy: A medical procedure involving the use of an endoscope to examine the inside of the nasal passages.

decongestants: Medications that relieve nasal congestion by narrowing the blood vessels in the nasal passages, making breathing easier.

humidifier: A machine that adds moisture to the air.

Vocabulary Challenge

1. The _____ in my face is becoming increasingly uncomfortable.
2. If you experience persistent _____, it may be a sign of a sinus infection.
3. A _____ is a machine that adds moisture to the air.
4. The doctor recommended a _____ to get a closer look inside my nasal passages.
5. _____ can help relieve nasal congestion by narrowing blood vessels in the nasal passages.
6. _____ is a common symptom of a cold or a sinus infection.
7. During a _____, a healthcare professional thoroughly examines the body to assess signs and symptoms.
8. _____ is inflammation or infection of the sinuses, commonly caused by bacteria, viruses, or allergies.

9. _____refers to pain or unease related to the teeth or gums.

Answers

1. pressure
2. symptoms
3. humidifier
4. nasal endoscopy
5. decongestants
6. nasal discharge
7. physical examination
8. sinus infection
9. dental discomfort

Comprehension Questions

1. What symptoms is the patient experiencing that suggest a possible sinus infection?
2. How long has the patient been dealing with the symptoms?
3. Initially, what did the patient think might be the cause of their symptoms?
4. Why did the patient decide to seek medical help?
5. What additional symptoms, besides congestion and nasal discharge, does the patient mention?
6. According to the doctor, what are common symptoms of a sinus infection?
7. What medical examinations does the doctor suggest to the patient?
8. If the patient indeed has a sinus infection, what does the doctor mention as part of the treatment plan?
9. Apart from medication, what home remedies does the doctor recommend?

Answers

1. The patient is experiencing symptoms such as congestion, constant pressure in the face, and nasal discharge.

2. The patient has been dealing with the symptoms for about a week.

3. Initially, the patient thought the cause of their symptoms might be a cold.

4. The patient decided to seek medical help because the symptoms haven't improved, and the pressure in the face is getting more uncomfortable.

5. Additional symptoms mentioned by the patient include headaches, especially around the forehead and eyes, and a reduced sense of smell.

6. According to the doctor, common symptoms of a sinus infection include facial pain, headaches, and a reduced sense of smell.

7. The doctor suggests a physical examination and a nasal endoscopy for the patient.

8. If the patient indeed has a sinus infection, the doctor mentions a treatment plan involving antibiotics, decongestants, and saline nasal irrigation.

9. Apart from medication, the doctor recommends home remedies such as warm compresses on the face, over-the-counter pain relievers, and using a humidifier.

Discussion Questions

1. In the dialogue, the patient initially thought they had a cold. Why might people mistake a sinus infection for a common cold, and what distinguishes the two?

2. What are your thoughts on combining medical treatments with home remedies for various health conditions?

3. How important do you think it is for individuals to seek medical help when experiencing persistent symptoms, as illustrated in the dialogue?

4. What are your views on the use of antibiotics, and do you think they are overprescribed in some cases?

5. How important do you think lifestyle factors, such as hydration and rest, are in managing and recovering from illnesses?

A Broken Arm

A patient suspects that she may have broken her arm.

Doctor: Good evening. I'm Dr. Smith. How can I assist you today?

Patient: Hi, Dr. Smith. I'm Lisa. I had a **fall**, and I think I might have broken my arm.

Doctor: Let's take a look. Can you describe how the injury occurred?

Patient: I tripped on the stairs at home and landed on my **outstretched** arm.

Doctor: I'm going to start by checking the **range of motion.** Can you try to move your fingers for me?

Patient: Ow, it hurts, but I can move them a bit.

Doctor: Alright. Let me take a look at your arm and assess the damage. I'll be gentle, but please let me know if it becomes too painful.

Doctor: Based on my initial examination, it seems like you might have a **fracture**. I'll order an X-ray to get a clearer picture. In the meantime, we'll give you something for the pain.

Patient: Okay, thank you. I'm a bit worried. How serious is it?

Doctor: Fractures can vary in **severity**, but we'll have a clearer understanding after the **X-ra**y. In the meantime, I'll arrange for a **splint** to help stabilize your arm.

Patient: That sounds good. Do I need a **cast**?

Doctor: We'll decide that based on the X-ray results. If it's a straightforward fracture, a cast might be necessary for proper healing. If it's more complex, you may need **surgery**.

Patient: Got it. How long does it usually take for a broken arm to heal?

Doctor: The healing time depends on the type and location of the fracture. I'll discuss a detailed treatment plan with you once we have the X-ray results.

Vocabulary

fall: To accidentally drop or descend to a lower position, often resulting in injury.

fracture: A break or crack in a bone, often caused by physical trauma.

outstretched: Extended or stretched out to its full length.

range of motion: The extent to which a joint can move in various directions.

x-ray: A diagnostic imaging technique that uses electromagnetic radiation to create images of the inside of the body, in this case, to visualize the bone.

splint: A device used to support and immobilize a broken or injured bone.

severity: The degree or extent of something.

cast: A rigid protective covering applied to a broken bone to aid in its healing and prevent movement.

surgery: Medical procedure involving incisions, manipulations, or repairs, often necessary for complex or severe fractures.

Vocabulary Challenge

1. After the _____ from the ladder, he suspected he might have a bone _____ in his arm.

2. The gymnast's _____ arm demonstrated the incredible flexibility of her joints.

3. The doctor recommended a(n) _____ to immobilize the fractured leg and promote healing.

4. The _____ revealed a clear image of the broken bone, helping the doctor make an accurate diagnosis.

5. The athlete's injury required _____ to repair the complex fracture in his ankle.

6. To aid in the healing process, the doctor applied a _____ to the patient's broken wrist.

7. The _____ of the injury was determined through a thorough examination and X-ray results.

8. The accident resulted in the _____ of his arm, making it necessary for medical intervention.

Answers

1. fall
2. outstretched
3. splint
4. x-ray
5. surgery
6. cast
7. severity
8. fracture

Comprehension Questions

1. Who is the doctor in the dialogue, and what is the patient's name?
2. How did Lisa injure herself, leading her to seek medical assistance?
3. What part of Lisa's body did she land on during the fall?
4. What is the doctor's first step in assessing Lisa's injury?
5. How does Lisa describe the pain when she attempts to move her fingers?
6. What does the doctor plan to do based on the initial examination of Lisa's arm?
7. What additional diagnostic tool does the doctor suggest to get a clearer picture of Lisa's injury?
8. How does the doctor reassure Lisa before proceeding with the examination?
9. What immediate measure does the doctor plan to take to address Lisa's pain?
10. How does the doctor respond when Lisa expresses concern about the seriousness of her injury?

Answers:

1. The doctor in the dialogue is Dr. Smith, and the patient's name is Lisa.

2. Lisa injured herself by tripping on the stairs at home, leading her to seek medical assistance.

3. Lisa landed on her outstretched arm during the fall.

4. The doctor's first step in assessing Lisa's injury is checking the range of motion, asking her to move her fingers.

5. Lisa describes the pain as, "Ow, it hurts, but I can move them a bit."

6. Based on the initial examination of Lisa's arm, the doctor plans to order an X-ray to get a clearer picture.

7. The additional diagnostic tool the doctor suggests to get a clearer picture of Lisa's injury is an X-ray.

8. Before proceeding with the examination, the doctor reassures Lisa by stating they will be gentle and asks her to inform if it becomes too painful.

9. The doctor plans to give Lisa something for the pain as an immediate measure.

10. In response to Lisa's concern about the seriousness of her injury, the doctor explains that fractures can vary in severity, and they'll have a clearer understanding after the X-ray. The doctor also mentions arranging for a splint to help stabilize Lisa's arm.

Discussion Questions

1. How important do you think it is for individuals to seek medical attention promptly after experiencing an injury or fall?

2. In what ways can accidents at home be prevented to reduce the risk of injuries like the one described in the dialogue?

3. In your opinion, what role does effective communication play in the doctor-patient relationship, especially in emergency situations?

4. How might the emotional state of a patient, like Lisa's worry, impact their experience and recovery process when facing a potential injury?

5. Share your thoughts on the balance between immediate pain relief measures and waiting for more detailed diagnostic results before determining a treatment plan.

6. Discuss the role of preventive measures, like splints and casts, in the overall treatment plan for fractures. How do these aids contribute to the healing process?

A Rash

A patient is talking to his doctor about a rash on his skin.

Patient: Good morning, Dr. Smith. I've been dealing with this skin **rash** for a few days, and it doesn't seem to be getting better.

Doctor: Good morning! I'm sorry to hear about your skin rash. Let's take a look. Can you describe the rash and when you first noticed it?

Patient: It started as a small red patch on my arm, but now it's spreading. It's itchy and a bit raised. I noticed it about a week ago.

Doctor: I see. Have you been using any new **skincare products** or **detergents** recently? Any changes in your diet or exposure to potential **allergens**?

Patient: No, I haven't changed anything in my **routine**.

Doctor: Alright. Any other symptoms accompanying the rash, like fever or pain?

Patient: No fever, but it's a bit **tender** to the touch. And the itching is getting worse.

Doctor: Let's rule out some possibilities. It could be an **allergic reaction,** contact dermatitis, or possibly a fungal infection. I'll need to take a closer look.

Patient: Sure, whatever it takes to get rid of this. It's really bothering me.

Doctor: I'll prescribe a **topical cream** to help with the **itching** and **inflammation**. Make sure to keep it clean and avoid scratching. We'll schedule a follow-up to discuss the test results.

Vocabulary

rash: A visible change in the skin's texture or color, often accompanied by itching or discomfort.

skincare products: Substances used for the care and maintenance of the skin.

detergents: Substances used for cleaning, especially laundry.

routine: A regular and consistent pattern of activities or behaviors.

allergens: Substances that can trigger an allergic reaction in some individuals.

inflammation: The body's response to injury or infection, characterized by redness, swelling, and pain.

tender: Sensitive or painful when touched.

itching: The sensation that prompts a desire to scratch the skin.

allergic reaction: The body's immune system response to a substance it considers harmful, resulting in symptoms like rash, itching, or swelling.

topical cream: A medication applied directly to the skin's surface for localized treatment.

Vocabulary Challenge

1. The _____ started as a small red patch on my arm, but now it's spreading. It's itchy and a bit raised.

2. _____ are substances used for the care and maintenance of the skin, such as lotions, creams, and cleansers.

3. I haven't changed anything in my _____.

4. _____ are substances used for cleaning, especially laundry or personal hygiene products.

5. _____ are substances that can trigger an allergic reaction in some individuals.

6. Let's rule out some possibilities. It could be an _____, contact dermatitis, or possibly a fungal infection.

7. No fever, but it's a bit _____ to the touch. And the _____ is getting worse.

8. _____ is the body's response to injury or infection, characterized by redness, swelling, and pain.

9. _____ is a medication applied directly to the skin's surface for localized treatment.

Answers:

1. rash
2. skincare products
3. routine
4. detergents
5. allergens
6. allergic reaction
7. tender; itching
8. inflammation
9. topical cream

Comprehension Questions

1. What is the patient's main concern when talking to the doctor?
2. How does the patient describe the rash initially?
3. How long has the patient been dealing with the skin rash?
4. When did the patient first notice the rash?
5. How does the patient describe the current state of the rash?
6. What changes has the patient made in their skincare routine or exposure to substances?
7. Are there any other symptoms accompanying the rash, according to the patient?
8. What possibilities does the doctor mention in relation to the rash?
9. What will the doctor do to further investigate the rash?
10. What does the doctor prescribe to help with the itching and inflammation?

Answers:

1. The patient's main concern is the skin rash not improving.

2. The patient describes the rash as starting as a small red patch on the arm and becoming itchy and raised.

3. The patient has been dealing with the skin rash for a few days.

4. The patient first noticed the rash about a week ago.

5. The patient describes the current state of the rash as spreading, itchy, and a bit raised.

6. The patient hasn't made any changes in their skincare routine or exposure to substances.

7. According to the patient, there is no fever, but the rash is tender to the touch, and the itching is getting worse.

8. The doctor mentions possibilities such as an allergic reaction, contact dermatitis, or a fungal infection.

9. The doctor will need to take a closer look to further investigate the rash.

10. The doctor prescribes a topical cream to help with the itching and inflammation.

Discussion Questions

1. How common are skin rashes, and what are some common causes?

2. How can individuals differentiate between a minor skin irritation and a more serious dermatological issue?

3. How does stress or mental health impact skin health, and vice versa?

4. Discuss the importance of proper skincare routines and the potential impact of using new skincare products.

5. Explore the psychological impact of skin issues and how it might affect a person's overall well-being.

Food Poisoning

*A patient is talking to the doctor about his **upset stomach**.*

Doctor: How can I help you today?

Patient: Hi, Doctor. I've been feeling really sick since yesterday. I think it might be something I ate.

Doctor: I'm sorry to hear that. Can you tell me more about your **symptoms**?

Patient: I've had stomach cramps, **nausea**, **vomiting**, and **diarrhea**.

Doctor: I'm sorry to hear that. It sounds like you might be experiencing **food poisoning**. Have you eaten anything unusual or from a different place recently?

Patient: Well, I did try a new restaurant a couple of days ago. I had some seafood, and that's when it all started.

Doctor: Seafood can sometimes be a **culprit**. Based on your symptoms, it seems likely.

Patient: What can I do about it?

Doctor: Firstly, we need to keep you **hydrated**. Drink plenty of fluids, and you might want to try **rehydration solutions**. I'll also **prescribe** some medication to help with the nausea.

Patient: Okay, thank you, Doctor. I just want to feel better.

Doctor: I understand. It usually takes a few days for the symptoms to improve, but if you notice any worsening or if you can't keep anything down, please come back to see me.

Vocabulary

upset stomach: A condition where the stomach feels uneasy.

symptoms: Indications or signs of a medical condition.

food poisoning: Illness caused by consuming contaminated food or beverages, leading to symptoms like nausea, vomiting, and diarrhea.

nausea: A sensation of unease and discomfort in the stomach.

vomiting: The act of expelling the contents of the stomach through the mouth.

diarrhea: The frequent passage of loose or watery stools.

culprit: The specific factor or substance responsible for causing harm or trouble.

rehydration solutions: Fluids containing electrolytes and nutrients to replenish lost fluids and minerals, often used to manage dehydration.

prescribe: To authorize the use of a specific medication or treatment for a patient.

hydrated: Maintaining an adequate level of bodily fluids.

Vocabulary Challenge

1. The doctor examined Mary's _____ and identified signs of dehydration and digestive issues.

2. Consuming contaminated water during the camping trip resulted in severe _____ for the entire group.

3. The _____ for the sudden illness was traced back to the undercooked meat at the family barbecue.

4. The physician decided to _____ antibiotics to help the patient recover from the bacterial infection.

5. Dehydration can be effectively managed with the use of _____, providing essential nutrients and fluids.

6. Experiencing an _____ after trying a new street food, Michael sought medical advice for relief.

7. The doctor advised the patient to stay _____ by drinking plenty of water throughout the day.

Answers

1. symptoms
2. food poisoning
3. culprit
4. prescribe
5. rehydration solutions
6. upset stomach
7. hydrated

Comprehension Questions

1. How does the patient describe their current state to the doctor?
2. What are the specific symptoms the patient mentions to the doctor?
3. What does the doctor suspect might be causing the patient's symptoms?
4. Where does the patient suspect they might have contracted their illness?
5. What did the patient eat a couple of days ago that might be related to their symptoms?
6. According to the doctor, what can sometimes be a culprit for the patient's symptoms?
7. What are the initial recommendations the doctor gives to the patient for managing their symptoms?
8. What does the doctor prescribe to help with the patient's nausea?
9. How long does the doctor suggest it might take for the patient's symptoms to improve?
10. What advice does the doctor give to the patient if their symptoms worsen or if they can't keep anything down?

Answers

1. The patient describes feeling really sick since yesterday.

2. The specific symptoms mentioned are stomach cramps, nausea, vomiting, and diarrhea.

3. The doctor suspects the patient might be experiencing food poisoning.

4. The patient suspects they might have contracted the illness from a new restaurant they tried a couple of days ago.

5. The patient ate seafood a couple of days ago, which might be related to their symptoms.

6. According to the doctor, seafood can sometimes be a culprit for the patient's symptoms.

7. The initial recommendations include staying hydrated, drinking plenty of fluids, and trying rehydration solutions. The doctor also prescribes medication to help with nausea.

8. The doctor prescribes medication to help with the patient's nausea.

9. The doctor suggests it usually takes a few days for the symptoms to improve.

10. The doctor advises the patient to come back if their symptoms worsen or if they can't keep anything down.

Discussion Questions

1. How can individuals reduce the risk of food poisoning when dining out?

2. Share personal experiences or stories about instances of food poisoning and discuss what measures could have been taken to prevent it.

3. Discuss the challenges individuals might face in staying hydrated when experiencing symptoms like nausea, vomiting, and diarrhea.

4. Explore the role of technology and social media in spreading awareness about food safety and preventing food borne illnesses.

5. Share tips and advice for people with an upset stomach.

Birth Control

A patient is talking to her doctor about birth control options.

Patient: I've been thinking about using birth control pills and wanted to discuss my options.

Doctor: Before we proceed, could you share a bit more about your medical history and if you've been on any form of birth control before?

Patient: Sure. I've never been on any birth control before. I'm generally healthy, and I don't have any medical issues.

Doctor: There are various types of **birth control pills** available, and we can discuss which might be the most suitable for you. Do you have any specific preferences?

Patient: I've heard about **combination pills** and **progestin-only pills**. I'm not sure which one would be better for me. Also, I'm a bit worried about potential side effects.

Doctor: Combination pills contain both estrogen and progestin, while progestin-only pills contain only progestin. We can explore both options and discuss the potential **side effects**. It's crucial to consider your **medical history** and any factors like smoking or certain health conditions that might influence the choice.

Patient: Okay. I'm a **non-smoker.** I want something effective and with minimal side effects.

Doctor: I'll explain how each type works, potential side effects, and how to take them correctly. We can discuss any potential **drug interactions** or factors that might affect their effectiveness.

Patient: Sounds good. Also, I've heard about **IUDs**. Should I consider that?

Doctor: They can be a good option for some people, but it depends on your preferences and lifestyle. We can certainly talk about them as well.

Patient: Okay, I appreciate that. I just want to make an **informed decision.**

Doctor: Absolutely. It's essential to consider your individual needs and preferences. We'll work together to find the right option for you.

Vocabulary

birth control pills: Medications taken orally to prevent pregnancy, with various types available.

medical history: A record of a person's past health conditions, surgeries, and medications.

combination pills: Birth control pills containing both estrogen and progestin hormones.

Progestin-only pills: Birth control pills containing only progestin hormone.

side effects: Unintended and often undesirable effects of a medication.

non-smoker: An individual who does not engage in the habit of smoking tobacco.

drug interactions: Effects that occur when the effects of one drug are altered by the presence of another drug.

IUD (intrauterine device): A small device that is placed inside the uterus to prevent pregnancy.

informed decision: A decision made with full awareness and understanding of the options, risks, and benefits involved.

Vocabulary Challenge

1. A _____ involves a record of a person's past health conditions, surgeries, and medications.

2. _____ are birth control pills containing both estrogen and progestin hormones.

3. _____ are birth control pills containing only progestin hormone.

4. _____ are unintended and often undesirable consequences of a medication.

5. An individual characterized as a _____ refrains from the habitual use of tobacco by smoking.

6. An _____, abbreviated as IUD, is a small device placed inside the uterus to prevent pregnancy.

7. An _____ is a decision made with full awareness and understanding of the options, risks, and benefits involved.

Answers:

1. medical history
2. combination pills
3. Progestin-only pills
4. side effects
5. non-smoker
6. intrauterine device
7. informed decision

Comprehension Questions

1. What is the patient's experience with birth control before this discussion?
2. What are the two types of birth control pills mentioned in the dialogue?
3. Why does the doctor emphasize the importance of considering the patient's medical history and lifestyle factors?
4. What does the patient mean when she says she's a non-smoker?
5. What does the doctor offer to discuss regarding the birth control pills?
6. Why does the patient express concern about potential side effects?
7. What additional birth control method does the patient inquire about?
8. How does the doctor respond to the patient's question about IUDs?
9. What is the patient's main goal in the conversation?
10. How does the doctor assure the patient that they will find the right option for her?

Answers

1. The patient has never been on any form of birth control before.

2. The two types of birth control pills mentioned are combination pills and progestin-only pills.

3. The doctor emphasizes considering the patient's medical history and lifestyle factors to determine the most suitable birth control option.

4. The patient is a non-smoker, meaning she does not smoke.

5. The doctor offers to discuss how each type of birth control pill works, potential side effects, and how to take them correctly.

6. The patient expresses concern about potential side effects because she's unsure which type of birth control pill would be better for her.

7. The patient inquires about IUDs (intrauterine devices).

8. The doctor states that IUDs can be a good option depending on the patient's preferences and lifestyle.

9. The patient's main goal is to make an informed decision about the suitable birth control option.

10. The doctor assures the patient that they will work together to find the right option for her individual needs and preferences.

Discussion Questions

1. How important do you think it is for individuals to have open and informed discussions with their healthcare providers about birth control options?

2. What are some common misconceptions or concerns people might have about birth control pills, and how can healthcare providers address them?

3. What are some advantages and disadvantages of IUDs as a birth control option?

4. What factors might influence an individual's decision to choose one type of birth control over another?

5. In your opinion, how can society contribute to promoting awareness and education about various birth control options?

A Physical Exam

Keith is getting an exam done by his doctor.

Doctor: When was the last time you came in for an exam?

Keith: I'm not sure. It's been a long time. Maybe two years.

Doctor: Okay, any problems that I should be aware of? Have you been feeling good?

Keith: No problems and I've been feeling pretty good, even though I just turned 50! I am taking **anti-depressants** though.

Doctor: I see. How's your mood now?

Keith: Much better since I started taking the medication.

Doctor: Okay, please **roll up your sleeve**. I'll take your **blood pressure**. That's good: **125/80**. And what about exercise? How often do you do it? And your diet?

Keith: Almost every day. I like to run and bike. I eat mostly **vegan** meals.

Doctor: I'm going to listen to your heart now. Okay. That sounds fine. I'm going to send you for a blood test to check your **cholesterol** and a few other things.

Vocabulary

anti-depressants: Medicine designed to help people who are depressed.

roll up your sleeve: What you need to do if you're getting a needle in your arm for a blood test, or getting your blood pressure taken. It means to lift (roll) up the arm on your shirt.

blood pressure: How much pressure your heart exerts pumping blood over the force your heart exerts in between beats.

125/80 (one twenty five over eighty): Systolic pressure of the heart (when it pumps or beats) over diastolic pressure (the force at rest).

vegan: Describes someone who doesn't consume animal products.

Vocabulary Challenge

1. Please _____ now. This will hurt a little bit.

2. I'm trying to make more _____ meals for my family but my teenage boys have been resisting me.

3. Your _____ is excellent for someone in their 80's.

4. Have you had your blood pressure checked lately? Oh, I think it's around _____.

5. I'm going to give you a prescription for some _____ and recommend a counsellor.

Answers

1. roll up your sleeve

2. vegan

3. blood pressure

4. 125/80

5. anti-depressants

Comprehension Questions

1. How long has it been since Keith's last exam?
2. Has Keith been experiencing any health problems, according to the information provided?
3. What is Keith's mood like since he started taking anti-depressants?
4. What is Keith's blood pressure reading during the examination?
5. How often does Keith engage in exercise, and what activities does he enjoy?
6. What type of meals does Keith mostly eat?
7. What additional test does the doctor plan to send Keith for?
8. Why does the doctor want to check Keith's cholesterol and other factors?
9. How does Keith describe his overall well-being during the exam?
10. Based on the information provided, does Keith seem generally healthy?

Answers

1. Keith last came in for an exam approximately two years ago.
2. Keith mentions that he has no problems and has been feeling pretty good, although he discloses taking anti-depressants.
3. He states that his mood has improved since he started taking the medication.
4. The doctor checks his blood pressure and reports it as 125/80.
5. Keith exercises almost every day, preferring activities like running and biking.
6. He follows a mostly vegan diet.
7. The doctor plans to send Keith for a blood test to check his cholesterol and other health markers.
8. The doctor wants to understand Keith's overall health and well-being.
9. Keith describes feeling pretty good in response to the doctor's inquiry about his mood.
10. Yes, he appears generally healthy based on the provided information.

Discussion Questions

1. How often do you think adults should go for a routine medical exam, and why?

2. In what ways can mood and mental health impact a person's overall well-being?

3. What lifestyle factors could contribute to good health?

4. How important is regular exercise and a balanced diet in maintaining overall health?

5. Discuss the significance of routine checks like blood pressure and cholesterol tests in preventive healthcare.

6. Do you think Keith's lifestyle choices, such as exercise and a vegan diet, are contributing positively to his health? Why or why not?

Antibiotic Prescription

Someone is talking to a pharmacist about their prescription.

Pharmacist: Good afternoon! How can I assist you today?

Patient: Hi, I'm Sarah. My doctor prescribed an antibiotic for me, and I'm here to pick it up.

Pharmacist: Thank you, Sarah. Let me pull up your prescription. Ah, here it is. Your doctor has **prescribed amoxicillin**. Have you taken this antibiotic before?

Patient: No, it's the first time. What should I know about it?

Pharmacist: Amoxicillin is an antibiotic used to treat bacterial infections. It's important to take the **full course** as prescribed by your doctor, even if you start feeling better before finishing the medication. Skipping doses may not fully eliminate the infection.

Patient: Got it. Are there any potential side effects I should be aware of?

Pharmacist: Like any medication, amoxicillin can have side effects. The most common ones include nausea, vomiting, diarrhea, and rash. If you experience severe side effects like difficulty breathing or swelling, seek **medical attention** immediately.

Patient: Okay, I'll keep an eye out for those. Should I take it with food?

Pharmacist: Yes, it's generally recommended to take amoxicillin with food to help reduce the risk of **stomach upset**. If you **miss a dose**, take it as soon as you remember, but if it's almost time for your next dose, skip the missed one.

Patient: Thanks for the advice.

Pharmacist: Remember that it's essential to finish the entire prescription, even if you start feeling better. If you have any **concerns** or if your symptoms persist, contact your doctor.

Patient: Thanks for all the information. I appreciate your help.

Vocabulary

prescribed: Ordered or recommended by a medical professional.

Amoxicillin: A type of antibiotic used to treat bacterial infections.

side effects: Unintended and often undesirable effects of a medication.

stomach upset: Discomfort or unease in the stomach, often associated with medication.

miss a dose: Not taking a prescribed dose of medication at the scheduled time.

full course: Completing the entire prescribed duration of medication.

medical attention: Seeking assistance or care from a healthcare provider, especially in the case of severe or concerning symptoms.

concerns: Any worries, doubts, or issues that the patient may have regarding their health or the prescribed medication.

Vocabulary Challenge

1. The doctor _____ an antibiotic to treat the infection.
2. _____ is commonly used to treat a variety of bacterial infections.
3. Before taking any medication, it's essential to be aware of potential _____.
4. If you experience _____ after taking the medicine, consult your healthcare provider.
5. It's crucial not to _____, as it may affect the effectiveness of the treatment.
6. Completing the _____ of antibiotics helps ensure the infection is fully treated.
7. If you have any _____ about the prescribed medication, discuss them with your doctor.
8. In case of severe symptoms, seek _____ promptly to address the issue.

Answers:

1. prescribed
2. Amoxicillin
3. side effects
4. stomach upset
5. miss a dose
6. full course
7. concerns
8. medical attention

Comprehension Questions

1. What medication did the doctor prescribe to Sarah?
2. Is this the first time Sarah is taking the prescribed antibiotic?
3. Why does the pharmacist emphasize taking the full course of the antibiotic?
4. What are some potential side effects of amoxicillin mentioned by the pharmacist?
5. How does the pharmacist recommend reducing the risk of stomach upset when taking amoxicillin?
6. What advice does the pharmacist give if a dose of amoxicillin is missed?
7. Why does the pharmacist stress the importance of finishing the entire prescription?
8. In case of severe side effects, what does the pharmacist suggest the patient should do?
9. How does the patient express gratitude to the pharmacist at the end of the conversation?
10. If the patient's symptoms persist or if they have concerns, what does the pharmacist recommend the patient should do?

Answers:

1. The doctor prescribed amoxicillin to Sarah.

2. Yes, it's the first time Sarah is taking the prescribed antibiotic.

3. The pharmacist emphasizes taking the full course of the antibiotic to ensure the infection is fully treated.

4. The pharmacist mentions that potential side effects of amoxicillin include nausea, vomiting, diarrhea, and rash.

5. The pharmacist recommends taking amoxicillin with food to help reduce the risk of stomach upset.

6. If a dose of amoxicillin is missed, the pharmacist advises taking it as soon as you remember, but if it's almost time for the next dose, skip the missed one.

7. The pharmacist stresses the importance of finishing the entire prescription to make sure the infection is fully treated.

8. In case of severe side effects, the pharmacist suggests seeking medical attention immediately.

9. The patient expresses gratitude by saying, "Thanks for all the information. I appreciate your help."

10. If the patient's symptoms persist or if they have concerns, the pharmacist recommends contacting the doctor.

Discussion Questions

1. Discuss the importance of patient education about prescribed medications. How does it impact adherence to treatment plans?

2. Share personal experiences or stories related to antibiotic use. What challenges or concerns have you faced or witnessed?

3. Explore the role of pharmacists in providing information and guidance to patients about their medications. How can pharmacists enhance patient understanding and compliance?

4. What measures can individuals take to minimize the risk of side effects when taking prescribed medications?

5. Discuss the potential consequences of not completing a full course of prescribed antibiotics. How does it impact individual health and public health?

6. Explore cultural or regional variations in attitudes toward antibiotic use and medical treatments. How do cultural factors influence healthcare practices?

Back Pain

A patient is talking to his doctor about back pain.

Patient: I've been experiencing **persistent** back pain lately, and it's starting to **affect** my daily activities.

Doctor: Good morning! I'm sorry to hear that. Let's discuss your back pain in more detail. Can you describe the pain, such as its **location**, **intensity**, and any specific **triggers**?

Patient: The pain is in my lower back, and it's a **dull**, **constant** ache. Sometimes, it gets sharper, especially when I bend or lift things.

Doctor: I see. How long have you been dealing with this back pain? Any recent incidents or changes in your routine that might be linked to it?

Patient: It's been going on for a few weeks now. I can't pinpoint a specific **incident,** but my job involves a lot of sitting, and I've noticed the pain getting worse recently.

Doctor: Okay. Besides the pain, have you experienced any other symptoms, such as numbness, tingling, or weakness in your legs?

Patient: No, not really. It's mainly the discomfort in my lower back.

Doctor: I'll conduct a physical examination to assess the **range of motion** and any signs of **inflammation** or muscle tension. Based on the results, we might consider additional diagnostic tests like X-rays or MRI. In the meantime, I recommend avoiding activities that worsen the pain, applying ice or heat, and over-the-counter pain relievers. We'll discuss further steps after the examination.

Vocabulary

persistent: Continuing or enduring over an extended period without interruption.

affect: To produce a change or influence on something.

location: The place or position where something is situated or occurs.

intensity: The degree or strength of a sensation, in this context, the severity of the pain.

triggers: Factors or events that initiate or exacerbate a reaction or condition.

dull: A type of pain characterized by a lack of sharpness or severity.

constant: Unchanging, remaining the same over time.

incident: An occurrence or event, especially one that may have an impact on the situation.

range of motion: The extent to which a joint or body part can be moved in various directions.

inflammation: The body's response to injury or infection, often involving redness, swelling, and pain.

Vocabulary Challenge

1. The _____ache in my lower back has been bothering me for weeks.
2. The recent change in my work routine seems to _____the frequency of my back pain.
3. The _____of the pain makes it difficult to concentrate on my daily activities.
4. _____like improper posture or heavy lifting can worsen my back pain.
5. The pain has been _____, and I can't find relief even with rest.
6. I can't pinpoint a specific _____that might be causing the back pain.
7. The _____of my discomfort is mainly in the lower back region.

Answers:

1. dull
2. affect
3. intensity
4. triggers
5. persistent
6. incident
7. location

Comprehension Questions

1. Where is the patient experiencing pain?
2. How does the patient describe the pain in terms of sensation?
3. What triggers make the pain sharper for the patient?
4. How long has the patient been dealing with back pain?
5. What aspects of the patient's job might be linked to the back pain?
6. Besides pain, what other symptoms does the doctor inquire about?
7. How does the patient describe the duration of the back pain?
8. What specific actions make the pain sharper for the patient?
9. What recommendations does the doctor give for managing the pain before further examination?
10. What additional diagnostic tests does the doctor mention based on the physical examination results?

Answers:

1. The patient is experiencing pain in their lower back.

2. The pain is described as a dull and constant ache, sometimes getting sharper, especially when bending or lifting things.

3. Specific triggers for the pain include bending or lifting things.

4. The patient has been dealing with back pain for a few weeks.

5. The pain has worsened recently, and the patient attributes it to their job, which involves a lot of sitting.

6. Besides the pain, the patient has not experienced other symptoms like numbness, tingling, or weakness in the legs.

7. The patient has been dealing with back pain for a few weeks.

8. The pain gets sharper, especially when bending or lifting things.

9. The doctor recommends avoiding activities that worsen the pain, applying ice or heat, and using over-the-counter pain relievers.

10. Additional diagnostic tests like X-rays or MRI are considered based on the results of the physical examination.

Discussion Questions

1. How can prolonged sitting or specific job requirements contribute to back pain, and what lifestyle changes might help alleviate it?

2. Discuss the importance of a thorough medical history in understanding and addressing a patient's back pain. What information might be crucial in this context?

3. How does the patient's description of the pain (dull, constant ache, sharper with certain movements) help the doctor in understanding the nature of the back pain?

4. Discuss the role of self-care measures, like applying ice or heat and over-the-counter pain relievers, in managing back pain.

5. Consider the psychological impact of persistent pain on a person's daily activities and overall well-being. How might it affect their quality of life and mental health?

Abdominal Pain

A patient is talking to a nurse and a doctor in the ER.

Patient: Excuse me, I'm experiencing severe **abdominal pain**, and I'm feeling really unwell. I think I need to see a doctor.

Nurse: Please take a seat, and I'll get a doctor to see you as soon as possible.

[After a few hours, the doctor enters the room.]

Doctor: Good evening, I'm Dr. Rodriguez. What seems to be the problem?

Patient: Hi, Doctor. I've been having intense abdominal pain for the past few hours. It started suddenly, and it's getting worse. I also feel **nauseous** and a bit **lightheaded**.

Doctor: I see. I'll need to ask you a few questions to better understand what might be going on. When did the pain start, and can you describe its nature?

Patient: It started about four hours ago, and it's a sharp pain in my lower abdomen. It's constant, and I haven't experienced anything like this before.

Doctor: Have you noticed any other symptoms, like fever, vomiting, or changes in your bowel movements?

Patient: No fever, but I have vomited a couple of times, and my last bowel movement was a bit unusual – diarrhea and very **watery**.

Doctor: I'll need to perform a physical examination to check for any signs of **tenderness** or **swelling** in your abdomen. I might also order some tests, such as **blood work** or **imaging,** to get a clearer picture. In the meantime, we'll provide you with something for the nausea.

Patient: Okay, Doctor. I appreciate your help. I'm just worried about the pain.

Doctor: I understand. We'll do our best to figure out what's causing the pain and provide you with the **appropriate treatment.**

Patient: Thank you, Doctor. I hope we can find out what's going on soon.

Vocabulary

abdominal pain: Sharp or intense discomfort in the region of the abdomen.

nauseous: Feeling the urge to vomit.

lightheaded: Feeling dizzy or having a sensation of light-headedness, often associated with a lack of blood flow to the brain.

tenderness: Pain or discomfort when pressure is applied to a specific area of the body.

swelling: Abnormal enlargement or puffiness of a body part.

blood work: Diagnostic tests involving the analysis of blood samples.

imaging: Diagnostic procedures, such as X-rays or scans, to visualize the internal structures of the body.

watery: Consisting of or resembling water; in this context, describing the nature of bowel movements.

appropriate treatment: Medical care tailored to address the specific symptoms or conditions identified through diagnosis.

Vocabulary Challenge

1. The patient complained of _____in the lower abdomen.

2. After taking the medication, the patient felt _____and had to lie down.

3. The patient felt _____after standing up.

4. The doctor observed _____when examining the injured area.

5. Severe _____of the ankle was noticed after the injury.

6. The physician ordered _____to analyze the patient's blood.

7. _____techniques were used to get a clear picture of the internal organs.

8. The patient reported _____bowel movements, indicating a potential issue.

9. The nurse administered the _____to alleviate the patient's symptoms.

Answers:

1. abdominal pain

2. nauseous

3. lightheaded

4. tenderness

5. swelling

6. blood work

7. imaging

8. watery

9. appropriate treatment

Comprehension Questions

1. What is the reason for the patient seeking medical attention in the ER?

2. How does the nurse respond to the patient's request to see a doctor?

3. Who is the doctor that eventually sees the patient, and what is the patient's description of their symptoms?

4. How long has the patient been experiencing abdominal pain, and how does the patient describe the nature of the pain?

5. Besides abdominal pain, what other symptoms does the patient mention during the conversation?

6. What does the doctor suggest in terms of further examinations and tests?

7. What unusual aspects of the patient's bowel movements does the doctor inquire about?

8. How does the patient feel about the pain, and what does the doctor say in response to their concerns?

9. What does the doctor mention about providing something for the patient's nausea?

10. What is the overall tone of the conversation between the patient, nurse, and doctor?

Answers:

1. The patient is seeking medical attention in the ER due to severe abdominal pain, feeling unwell, and the need to see a doctor.

2. The nurse asks the patient to take a seat, assuring them that a doctor will see them as soon as possible.

3. The doctor who sees the patient is Dr. Rodriguez. The patient describes intense abdominal pain, nausea, and lightheadedness.

4. The patient has been experiencing abdominal pain for the past four hours. The pain is sharp, located in the lower abdomen, constant, and different from previous experiences.

5. The patient mentions vomiting and a recent unusual bowel movement (diarrhea with very watery stool) in addition to abdominal pain.

6. The doctor suggests a physical examination to check for tenderness or swelling in the abdomen and mentions the possibility of ordering tests such as blood work or imaging.

7. The doctor inquires about any changes in bowel movements, specifically asking about diarrhea and very watery stool.

8. The patient expresses worry about the pain, and the doctor acknowledges the concern, assuring the patient that they will do their best to figure out the cause and provide appropriate treatment.

9. The doctor mentions providing something for the patient's nausea while further examinations and tests are planned.

10. The overall tone of the conversation is professional and focused on addressing the patient's symptoms and concerns.

Discussion Questions

1. What are some common reasons why people might visit the emergency room?

2. How important is the initial interaction with the nurse when a patient arrives at the ER?

3. In what situations might abdominal pain be considered a medical emergency?

4. What challenges might healthcare professionals face when dealing with patients experiencing severe pain and discomfort?

5. How do you think patients feel when they have to wait for several hours in the ER before seeing a doctor?

6. What factors contribute to a positive or negative patient experience in the emergency room?

Talking About Lifestyle Changes

Allen is talking to his doctor about some bad test results.

Allen: So what's the news doc?

Dr. Qi: Well, it's bad news. The results show **high cholesterol** and that you're **pre-diabetic**.

Allen: Oh no. Is there some medication for that?

Dr. Qi: Yes, but let's talk about your lifestyle first. Do you smoke or **drink**?

Allen: Yes, **a pack a day** usually. And I have **a 6-pack** every night usually.

Dr. Qi: And what about exercise?

Allen: What's that? Hahaha!

Dr. Qi: And finally, how about your **diet**?

Allen: Well, bacon is my favorite food and I don't like vegetables that much.

Dr. Qi: Okay. Well, that explains the high cholesterol. Let's talk about some **lifestyle changes** in those areas before getting you on medication.

Vocabulary

high cholesterol: A type of fat found in the blood that comes from eating animal products.

pre-diabetic: Blood sugar levels are higher than they should be.

drink: Consume alcohol (a verb in this case).

a pack a day: Smoking an entire package of cigarettes every day.

a 6-pack: 6 cans of beer that are sold together in a package.

diet: Food you eat.

lifestyle changes: Making changes regarding smoking, drinking, sleeping, diet, etc.

Vocabulary Challenge

1. You'll need to make some _____ if you want to avoid type 2 diabetes.

2. I had _____ so I adopted a vegan diet.

3. Wow! Ted likes to _____.

4. Let's pick up _____ for the party tonight.

5. What's your _____ like? Do you eat a lot of fruits and vegetables?

6. I'm _____ so am drastically changing my diet.

7. My brother smokes _____. I'm so worried about him.

Answers:

1. lifestyle changes

2. high cholesterol

3. drink

4. a 6-pack

5. diet

6. pre-diabetic

7. a pack a day

Comprehension Questions

1. What are Allen's test results indicating?

2. How much does Allen smoke daily?

3. How much does Allen drink every night?

4. What is Allen's attitude towards exercise?

5. How does Allen describe his diet preferences?

6. What lifestyle factors does Dr. Qi inquire about?

7. Why does Dr. Qi mention the need for lifestyle changes before medication?

8. What does Allen's favorite food contribute to, according to Dr. Qi?

9. In what order does Dr. Qi address different aspects of Allen's lifestyle?

Answers:

1. Allen received bad news about his health.

2. Allen mentioned that he smokes a pack a day.

3. Allen revealed that he typically consumes a 6-pack of alcohol every night.

4. Allen humorously stated that he doesn't know what exercise is.

5. Allen confessed that bacon is his favorite food, and he doesn't like vegetables.

6. The doctor inquired about smoking, drinking, exercise, and diet.

7. The doctor aims to address the root causes of Allen's health issues.

8. Allen is diagnosed with high cholesterol.

9. The doctor is exploring Allen's smoking and drinking habits, exercise routine, and dietary preferences.

Discussion Questions

1. What are some common lifestyle factors that can contribute to health issues?

2. How do smoking and excessive alcohol consumption impact overall health, and what changes could be made to improve these habits?

3. In what ways does regular exercise contribute to a healthy lifestyle, and how can individuals incorporate it into their routines?

4. What role does diet play in maintaining good health, and how can individuals make healthier food choices?

5. Why might a doctor recommend lifestyle changes before resorting to medication for certain health conditions?

6. What challenges might individuals face when trying to make significant lifestyle changes, and how can they overcome these challenges?

A High Fever

A parent is talking to a nurse about her daughter.

Parent: I'm really concerned about my daughter. She has a high **fever.**

Nurse: Can you tell me more about your child's **symptoms** and how high her fever is?

Parent: She's been feeling warm since yesterday, and her temperature is around 101 degrees Fahrenheit. She seems tired and has a bit of a cough.

Nurse: I'm sorry to hear that. It's essential to monitor her temperature regularly. Have you given her any fever-reducing medication, like **Acetaminophen** or **Ibuprofen**?

Parent: Yes, I gave her Acetaminophen, but her fever isn't going down.

Nurse: It's good that you've given her medication. If the fever persists, it might be best to bring her in for an examination. In the meantime, make sure she stays **hydrated**. Is she drinking enough fluids?

Parent: She's not interested in drinking, but I'm encouraging her to have some juice.

Nurse: If her condition doesn't improve or if you notice any concerning symptoms, such as difficulty breathing or persistent vomiting, it's crucial to seek medical attention promptly. Additionally, keep an eye on her overall behavior and **responsiveness.**

Parent: Thank you for the advice. I'm just worried because she's usually very active, and this fever is making her feel so **lethargic.**

Nurse: It's understandable to be concerned. Fevers can be common with **viral infections,** so it's essential to monitor her closely. If her symptoms persist or worsen, don't hesitate to reach out or visit the doctor.

Vocabulary

fever: A higher-than-normal body temperature, often a sign of illness or infection.

symptoms: Indications or signs of a medical condition, such as fever, cough, or tiredness.

Acetaminophen: A common over-the-counter medication used to reduce fever and pain.

Ibuprofen: Another over-the-counter medication, often used for reducing inflammation.

lethargic: Feeling sluggish, tired, or lacking in energy.

hydrated: Having an adequate amount of fluid in the body, often referring to staying well-hydrated by drinking fluids.

viral infections: Infections caused by viruses, which can lead to symptoms like fever, cough, and fatigue.

responsiveness: Reacting appropriately or showing a response to external stimuli, such as questions or treatment.

Vocabulary Challenge

1. A _____ is a higher-than-normal body temperature, often a sign of illness or infection.
2. _____ are indications or signs of a medical condition, such as fever, cough, or tiredness.
3. _____ is a common over-the-counter medication used to reduce fever and pain.
4. _____ is another over-the-counter medication, often used for reducing inflammation.
5. Feeling sluggish, tired, or lacking in energy is described as _____.
6. _____ refers to having an adequate amount of fluid in the body, often achieved by drinking fluids.
7. _____ are infections caused by viruses, which can lead to symptoms like fever, cough, and fatigue.
8. _____ is the term for reacting appropriately or showing a response to external stimuli, such as questions or treatment.

Answers:

1. fever
2. symptoms
3. Acetaminophen
4. Ibuprofen
5. lethargic
6. hydrated
7. viral infections
8. responsiveness

Comprehension Questions

1. What is the parent's primary concern regarding her daughter?
2. How long has the daughter been feeling warm, and what is her current temperature?
3. What symptoms does the daughter exhibit besides the fever?
4. What fever-reducing medications does the nurse mention, and which one did the parent give her daughter?
5. Despite giving Acetaminophen, what concern does the parent express about the daughter's fever?
6. What does the parent need to do if the daughter's fever persists?
7. What advice does the nurse give regarding the daughter's fluid intake?
8. Why does the nurse emphasize monitoring for symptoms like difficulty breathing or persistent vomiting?
9. How does the parent describe the daughter's usual behavior, and how is it affected by the fever?
10. What does the nurse suggest about fevers and viral infections, and what action does she recommend if symptoms persist or worsen?

Answers:

1. The parent's primary concern is her daughter's high fever.

2. The daughter has been feeling warm since yesterday, and her temperature is around 101 degrees Fahrenheit.

3. Besides the fever, the daughter is tired and has a bit of a cough.

4. The nurse mentions Acetaminophen and Ibuprofen, and the parent gave her daughter Acetaminophen.

5. Despite giving Acetaminophen, the parent expresses concern that the daughter's fever isn't going down.

6. If the daughter's fever persists, the nurse suggests bringing her in for an examination.

7. The nurse advises making sure the daughter stays hydrated.

8. The nurse emphasizes monitoring for symptoms like difficulty breathing or persistent vomiting because they may indicate a more serious condition.

9. The parent describes the daughter as usually very active, but the fever is making her feel lethargic.

10. The nurse suggests that fevers can be common with viral infections, and she recommends reaching out or visiting the doctor if symptoms persist or worsen.

Discussion Questions

1. What role does hydration play in managing a child's illness?

2. In what ways can a parent balance home care and seeking medical attention?

3. What might be the emotional and practical challenges for a parent when a usually active child becomes lethargic due to illness?

4. Discuss the significance of recognizing symptoms like difficulty breathing or persistent vomiting and taking prompt action.

5. How might the parent's worry about the daughter's deviation from her usual activity level impact the overall caregiving approach and decision-making process?

Before You Go

If you found this book useful, please leave a review wherever you bought it. It will help other English learners, like yourself find this resource.

Please send me an email with any questions or feedback that you might have.

YouTube: www.youtube.com/c/jackiebolen

Pinterest: www.pinterest.com/eslspeaking

ESL Speaking: www.eslspeaking.org

Email: jb.business.online@gmail.com

You might also be interested in these books (by Jackie Bolen):

- Short Stories in English for Intermediate Learners

- Master English Collocations in 15 Minutes a Day

- IELTS Academic Vocabulary Builder

Please also join my email list. You'll get helpful tips, ideas and resources for learning English, delivered straight to your inbox each week: www.eslspeaking.org/learn-english.

Made in the USA
Las Vegas, NV
22 November 2024

12389325R00059